Childhood Apraxia of Speech Resource Guide

SINGULAR RESOURCE GUIDE SERIES

EDITOR

Ken M. Bleile, Ph.D.
Department of Communicative Disorders
University of Northern Iowa
Cedar Falls, Iowa

ASSOCIATE EDITORS

Brian Goldstein, Ph.D.
Communication Sciences
Temple University
Philadelphia, Pennsylvania

Sharon Glennen, Ph.D.
Department of Communication
Sciences and Disorders
Towson University
Towson, Maryland

Carole Roth, Ph.D.
Department of Speech Pathology
Hennepin County Medical Center
Minneapolis, Minnesota

Amy Weiss, Ph.D
Department of Speech Pathology and Audiology
University of Iowa
Iowa City, Iowa

Tricia Zebrowski, Ph.D.
Department of Speech Pathology and Audiology
University of Iowa
Iowa City, Iowa

Childhood Apraxia of Speech Resource Guide

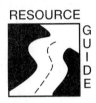

RESOURCE GUIDE

Shelley L. Velleman, Ph.D., CCC/SLP
Communication Disorders
University of Massachusetts–Amherst

THOMSON

DELMAR LEARNING

Australia Canada Mexico Singapore Spain United Kingdom United States

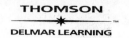

THOMSON

DELMAR LEARNING

Childhood Apraxia of Speech Research Guide
by Shelley L. Velleman, Ph.D., CCC/SLP

Executive Director, Health Care Business Unit:
William Brottmiller

Executive Editor:
Cathy L. Esperti

Acquisitions Editor:
Candice Janco

Developmental Editor:
Patricia Gaworecki

Editorial Assistant:
Maria D'Angelico

Executive Marketing Manager:
Dawn F. Gerrain

Channel Manager:
Jennifer McAvery

Production Editor:
James Zayicek

For permission to use material from this text or product, contact us by
Tel (800) 730-2214
Fax (800) 730-2215
www.thomsonrights.com

Library of Congress Catalog Card Number:

Velleman, Shelley Lynne.
    Childhood Apraxia of Speech Resource Guide / Shelley L. Velleman.
        p. cm.
    Includes index.
    ISBN 0-7693-0165-7
    1. Apraxia. 2. Motor ability in children. 3. Movement disorders in children. I. Title.

RJ496.A63 V455 2002
618.92'8552—dc21   2002023439

NOTICE TO THE READER

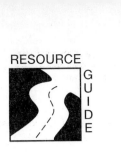

CONTENTS

ABOUT THE AUTHOR

Shelley L. Velleman, Ph.D., CCC-SLP is an assistant professor in the Communication Disorders Department at the University of Massachusetts at Amherst. She has a bachelor's degree from Wellesley College, master's degrees from the University of Wisconsin–Madison and the University of Massachusetts at Amherst, and a doctorate from the University of Texas at Austin. Her intellectual passion is child phonology—both normal and disordered. She approaches this field through the marriage of two perspectives: one provided by many years of direct clinical work, and the other by her Ph.D. in Linguistics. Thus, one of her major goals is to make theory both accessible and functional for practicing speech-language pathologists. She has been assessing, treating, and studying childhood apraxia of speech for over a decade.

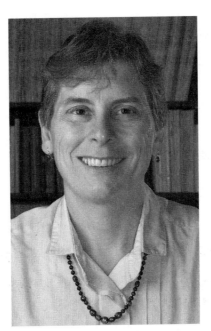

Source: Thom Kelly/UMass Creative Services

FOREWORD

The emblem for this series is a stylized road ending in an arrow. This symbol is intended to represent the goal of the series: to create books that serve as road maps to the care of communicative disorders. Like good road maps, each book gives the clinician an honest depiction of the territory, shows the various routes, and allows you the traveler to select the route best suited for your particular type of journey. Each book author is someone who knows the territory about which he or she is writing, both as a clinician and a researcher. The editorial board that advises the editors and authors is composed of some of the most respected persons in our profession. The hope of all involved in the series is that you will find the books useful and readable. Good traveling!

Ken Bliele, Ph.D.
Series Editor

PREFACE

I spent yesterday morning participating in the evaluation of a 3-year-old with a possible diagnosis of childhood apraxia of speech. The diagnosis had been tentatively raised a year ago, as a possibility that could not be ruled out because the child, at 25 months, was then speaking only a few words. Since that time, this little girl had made remarkable progress, and was now speaking in five-word, mostly intelligible sentences. Because some of her substitution patterns were unusual (e.g., [v] inconsistently substituted for /w/ and for liquid clusters), ongoing speech-language therapy was definitely warranted. However, she exhibited no signs of oral or speech apraxia. Yet neither the speech-language pathologist who had worked with her over the past year nor a speech-language pathologist at another clinic who had done a second-opinion evaluation in the meantime was confident enough to rule out an apraxia diagnosis completely.

We are currently faced with a dilemma with respect to childhood apraxia of speech: the label is being given increasingly to a growing number of children with various sorts of phonological delays and disorders. Yet many of those who work with these children, including some who mention the possibility of this diagnosis to parents, are insecure in their knowledge and skills for identifying and treating childhood apraxia of speech. This is not the fault of the practicing speech-language pathologist; it reflects two problems. First, there is a sorry lack of information about this disorder. Furthermore, the published information that is available is often contradictory and almost completely based upon the clinical experience of the authors, rather than on actual studies of treatment efficacy. Thus, while the procedures they recommend may be effective, we do not know whether they are efficient (i.e., maximally effective within the shortest possible treatment time). Second, the published information that is available typically focuses on theory, with only very general suggestions for assessment and treatment. Specific procedures have to be inferred by busy professionals with little time to read between the lines.

This *Childhood Apraxia of Speech Resource Guide* does not provide answers to the myriad questions that remain to be addressed through clinical research; those answers are not yet available. Neither is it completely devoid of bias; it is based upon this author's experience and critical reading of the research and clinical materials available. However, it is an attempt to address the second problem: to gather together what has been learned thus far about childhood apraxia of speech into a concrete, practical, comprehensive guide that the practicing speech-language pathologist can use as a resource to aid in day-to-day diagnostic and intervention decision making about children with possible childhood apraxia of speech. The many summaries and tables are intended to make the relevant information easily accessible and usable for the busy pediatric speech-language pathologist. The summaries are concise, but not lacking in detail. They list specific components of assessment and treatment approaches, with notes comparing more traditional approaches to those that are current today. Some tables include vital normative information about prelinguistic vocal development and the development of word and syllable shapes as well as of consonants and vowels. Additional tables facilitate documentation of these developments in particular clients with childhood apraxia of speech, as well as of communicative intents and means, communicative effectiveness, the prevalence of homonyms, and levels of inconsistency in children with apraxia. All technical terms are carefully defined, with examples, both in the text and in the glossary. My over-reaching goal in writing this guide has been to provide easily accessible information about *what to do* and *why*. It is my hope that it will increase your knowledge, skills, confidence, and efficiency as you work with this very challenging population.

This resource guide is divided into four main sections. The first section, *Core Knowledge*, is the most like a traditional textbook, providing definitions, perspectives, and some history of the study of childhood apraxia of speech. The next two sections, *Assessment* and *Treatment*, present information in more quickly accessible forms: summaries of assessment and treatment approaches, step-by-step procedures, normative tables, and clinical tables. Each begins with an overview of the content. Many of the topics in these sections begin with a box introducing the purpose and content of that topic, in the form of answers to a set of wh-questions:

> - WHO? Denotes for whom this topic is relevant (e.g., speech-language pathologists working with school-age children with possible childhood apraxia of speech).
>
> - WHAT? Denotes the theme of the topic (e.g., reading readiness and literacy).
>
> - WHY? Denotes the importance of the topic (e.g., the increased risk for literacy difficulties among children with childhood apraxia of speech).
>
> - LITERATURE RESOURCES: Lists references particularly relevant to the topic.

Section Four is a set of case studies, illustrating some of the thorny clinical issues that arise in children with this disorder, with discussion of assessment results and intervention strategies for each child. Long-term outcomes are presented where available.

The book also includes resources for the reader: bibliographies of electronic resources and suggested books for young children with childhood apraxia of speech, a key to the IPA symbols used in the book, a glossary of technical terms used in the book, and references.

Shelley L. Velleman
University of Massachusetts–Amherst

ACKNOWLEDGMENTS

My good friend and frequent collaborator Kristine Strand is directly or indirectly responsible for many of the ideas in this book. Her friendship and her intellectual stimulation have been precious to me ever since we first met at a job interview in 1984 or so—for a job I soon realized I didn't want and she soon realized she wouldn't offer me! I have also learned an enormous amount from other apraxia collaborators, including Larry Shriberg, Babs Davis, Ruth Bahr, Mary Andrianopoulos, and Diana Gonzalez.

All of the children and all of the parents, from little Eric on, have provided another invaluable source of intellectual excitement and inspiration. I have had the privilege, joy, and wonder of participating in the linguistic and social growth of scores of children—some directly in clinics at North Shore Children's Hospital, Weldon Center, Baystate Medical Center, and here at the University of Massachusetts, and some electronically, through the Childhood Apraxia of Speech Association of North America (CASANA) and its indomitable founder, Sharon Gretz. They are the real "bottom line."

Many other people were instrumental, in many different ways, in bringing this project to its completion. Amy Weiss, Patricia Gaworecki, Ken Bleile, Marie Linville, Kristin Banach, an anonymous reviewer, and my wonderfully detail-oriented unofficial editorial assistant Courtney Bolser provided very valuable input, feedback, and encouragement. My colleagues and students at the University of Massachusetts, especially Harry Seymour, Neva Frumkin, Lauren Bell, Lisa Hannahan, Caro Lambert, Sally-Anne Dunn, Tiffany Charko, Alyson Marcello, Manisha Shetty, Heidi Cahoon, and many others supported me, listened to my ideas, and asked hard questions about apraxia to keep me thinking. My very dear friends Babs Davis, Carol Stoel-Gammon, and Marilyn Vihman and of course my family, especially Dan, helped me to remember that there is life beyond apraxia and generally kept me sane.

Thank you all.

SECTION

CORE KNOWLEDGE

....

WHAT IS APRAXIA?

The short answer to this question is that **apraxia** is a lack of **praxis**. What, then, is praxis? Ayres (1985) defines it as "that neurological process by which cognition directs motor action, . . . the ability to formulate or plan different actions that allow the individual to affect the relationship between self and the environment [which] . . . occurs before actual motor execution" (p. 23). She emphasizes that a movement pattern is not simply a series of postures. It is critical for a motor plan to include information about the sequencing of these postures. Furthermore, sequencing postures does not consist simply of determining their order of occurrence. Even more critical to praxis, that is, motor planning, is the determination of how the articulators (or other body parts) will transition from one posture to the next. This involves a fine-tuned awareness of the current state and the desired future state of the articulators at any given moment, and a plan for smoothly transitioning from one state to the next. In other words, in Ayres's view, praxis is the generation of volitional movement patterns, including the selection, planning, organization, and initiation of the motor pattern. The execution of the motor pattern is merely the result of praxis, the overt manifestation of a successful, invisible process.

WHAT IS CHILDHOOD APRAXIA?

Childhood apraxia of speech is a condition that is estimated to occur in about one to 10 children per 1,000 (Shriberg, Aram, & Kwiatkowski, 1997a), a small proportion of the approximately 5% (five per 100) of children with phonological/articulatory disorders of

Clinical Note

It is important to note that the words "apraxia" and "**dyspraxia**" tend to be used interchangeably in the field of communication disorders, ignoring the etymological implication that *a*praxia (lack of praxis) is more severe than *dys*praxia (impaired praxis). In this book we will use the word "apraxia," the phrase "**childhood apraxia of speech**," and the acronym **CAS**. Further discussion on the question of what to call this disorder is provided in a later part of this section.

any kind. According to the 2001 American Speech-Language-Hearing Association Omnibus Survey (ASHA, 2001), 97.5% of school speech-language pathologists reported having an average of 23 children with articulation or phonological disorders on their caseloads at any given time; 74.7% of them stated that their caseloads include about four children with **dysarthria** or apraxia. Thus, about 17% of the typical school-setting therapist's articulation/phonology caseload is made up of children with motor speech disorders of some sort (dyspraxia or dysarthria). Part of the reason that these two disorders are lumped together on surveys is that the differentiation between the two (and also between apraxia and other phonological disorders) is murky in many people's minds. The answer to the question, "What is childhood apraxia?" is neither simple nor agreed-upon. Specialists in the field continue to disagree, for example, about whether a distinction should be made between motor apraxia and verbal apraxia. (This issue will be discussed further below.)

The vast majority of definitions of childhood apraxia of speech have included the idea of a motor-planning disorder in the absence of motor weakness. In this sense, apraxia is clearly differentiated from dysarthria. In dysarthria, the muscles themselves are affected with respect to their strength and **muscle tone**. If muscle tone is low, as in ataxic cerebral palsy, the muscles do not contract enough; they appear to be very loose and the person's movements are often unsteady. If muscle tone is high, the muscles contract too much, and the person's movements may appear to be very stiff. If tone is variable, as in athetoid type cerebral palsy, the muscle contractions are as well, resulting in involuntary movements. In dysarthria, these symptoms are quite independent of the context. Whether the person is attempting a well-learned activity, such as brushing her teeth or saying "good morning," or a more complex or novel activity, such as curling her tongue or repeating a multisyllabic nonsense word, the symptoms and their severity are the same. A person with dysarthria of speech can be expected to demonstrate reduced accuracy in all utterances, resulting in consonant cluster reduction, syllable omission, consonant distortion, and so on, in a pattern that is consistent across contexts. Thus, mispronunciations are quite predictable: complex sounds or sequences are difficult, regardless of the context, and are likely to be simplified or approximated.

Errors observed in apraxia, on the other hand, are not attributable to primary motor or sensory difficulties (Strub & Black, 1981). Furthermore, although some children with apraxia do exhibit mildly reduced muscle tone or sensory hypo- or hypersensitivity, the children's speech-language deficits are more significant than can be accounted for by these mild sensory or motor factors (Crary, 1984). In apraxia, the context makes a marked difference in the person's ability to perform. Actually brushing one's teeth, for example, is an overlearned, automatic activity, and is typically unimpaired. However, *pretending* to brush one's teeth may be very difficult. Although it is similar, the movement pattern is not identical to the automatic one and must therefore be generated anew, a much greater processing demand for the motor-planning system. Similarly, using a well-known word in an appropriate context versus repeating a nonsense word of the same phonetic difficulty level are very different tasks for the person with apraxia. In both of these cases, one version of the activity is **automatic**—so well-learned that no motor planning is required; an existing motor plan can be recruited. The other version of the activity, while no more difficult from the point of view of the muscle contractions required, is **volitional**—deliberate, not automatic, and therefore it depends upon planning a sequence of motor commands. This is where the difficulty lies: not in carrying out the motor commands, but in identifying the motor commands to be given, their order, and the transitions from one articulatory or other posture to the next.

Netsell (1981) tells us that spatio-temporal coordination dominates the development of speech motor control during the first six years of life, and that there is a gradual increase in overall execution speed of motor programs between the ages of 3 and 11 years. One of the last refinements to be perfected by young children is the conditioning or adaptation of segment durations according to the linguistic content of the utterance (length, complexity, etc.). Spatio-temporal coordination appears to be a specific area of deficit in childhood apraxia, with other aspects of motor control developing normally. This holds true for all types of apraxia, whether they affect motor planning for the mouth, the limbs, or the entire body.

The distinction between childhood apraxia of speech and other types of phonological disorders is less clear-cut and more debated. Opinions range from referring to childhood apraxia as "just another motor problem" (Robin, 1992, p. 19) to defining it as a centrally sensorimotor-based phonological disorder that impacts upon speech motor learning (Crary, 1984). In other words, some see childhood apraxia as a motor planning problem only, while others see it as phonological, or even more generally linguistic, *as well as motor*. The phonological nature of the disorder is seen in non-speech phonological symptoms, such as difficulties identifying rhymes and syllables (Marion, Sussman, & Marquardt, 1993; Marquardt, Sussman, Snow, & Jacks, 2002). The more generally linguistic nature of the disorder is seen in language symptoms, such as the mis-sequencing of words or morphemes within an utterance. Ekelman and Aram (1983) state unequivocally that "these children without exception also are presenting syntactic difficulties that cannot be attributed to motor speech restrictions alone" (p. 238). In addition, there may be subtle auditory processing difficulties (Bridgeman & Snowling, 1988), some of which may not be evident until the middle elementary school years. There is general agreement that symptoms of language and literacy learning difficulties often co-occur with childhood apraxia. The disagreement lies in the question of whether these symptoms (1) are symptoms inherent to the disorder (the linguistic or phonological view), (2) are unrelated effects of the brain differences that are presumed to be present (although they have yet to be identified) in children who have apraxia (the motor view), or (3) are the result of decreased experience with language and phonology due to production difficulties associated with apraxia.

There are many different labels given to this disorder, generally reflecting the views of those who use each label. Thus, proponents of a more motoric view of the disorder tend to refer to it as **developmental apraxia of speech (DAS)**. Those who believe that the phonological and language symptoms that tend to co-occur with the motor-planning symptoms are an inherent part of the disorder tend to use the label **developmental verbal dyspraxia (DVD)**. In both cases, the use of the word "developmental" has unfortunate practical implications: some insurance companies refuse to cover speech-language therapy for the disorder under these names because they believe that developmental disorders are those that will naturally improve over time without intervention. Recently, the Childhood Apraxia of Speech Association of North America (CASANA; further information available at http://www.apraxia.org) has advocated the more theory-neutral, insurance-friendly term **"childhood apraxia of speech."** This term, and its acronym (**CAS**), will be used throughout this book.

A related question is whether childhood apraxia is a **unitary disorder**, presenting with a single list of symptoms, or a **syndrome**. In a syndrome, a variety of symptoms—with a common underlying deficit—may or may not be present to different degrees in individual children with apraxia. Aram (1984) argues for the **symptom complex** view, stating that the symptoms include a phonological disorder, an expressive syntactic disorder, and variable articulatory patterns and neurological signs. Similarly, Crary (1993) proposes a continuum of symptoms associated with CAS, ranging from those that are very motoric (**executive apraxia**) to those that are more ideational and linguistic (**planning apraxia**). Velleman and Strand (1994) propose a common underlying deficit uniting the various (executive and planning) symptoms of the disorder that they term "developmental verbal dyspraxia" (DVD). In their view, children with CAS present with different symptoms, and these symptoms change over time in each individual. The underlying deficit is present in all those with childhood apraxia; with appropriate intervention, however, its manifestations may become undetectable in the long run. As Velleman and Strand describe it,

> the theory of "nonlinear phonology" emphasizes the hierarchical nature of phonological organization: phrases within sentences, words within phrases, groups of sounds (syllables, clusters, etc.) and/or morphemes within words, individual sounds within groups or morphemes; phrase stress and intonation within sentence stress and intonation, word stress within phrase stress, and so forth. [See box.] Another recent, more biologically-based model of phonology suggests that phonology and syntax share a "frame-content" organization, with syllable structure as the frame for sound segments, and grammar (including function words) as the frame for content words in sentences. These two models share the concept of linguistic units at different levels within a **hierarchy** that are organized for the processing and production of speech.
>
> Thus, children with DVD could be seen as impaired in their ability to generate and/or utilize hierarchical **frames**, which would otherwise provide the mechanisms for analyzing, organizing, and utilizing information from their motor, sensory and linguistic systems for the production of spoken language. This would account for the fact that children with DVD are often better able to produce sounds in isolation than in the context of a whole word, and that they are often better able to produce words in isolation than to assemble them into sentences. . . . From a linguistic standpoint, children with DVD might "have" the appropriate phonological (or syntactic) elements, but be unable to organize them into an appropriate cognitive hierarchy. Without the proper hierarchical representation of the action, an appropriate motor plan could not be devised. The lack of a hierarchical frame into which elements of action could be organized would account for the transition difficulties that are noted in reports of all forms of apraxia.
>
> . . . Thus, one might propose that the underlying source of the symptoms manifested in DVD is difficulty with "on-line" planning or programming of elements

of the language/speech system into larger organized patterns. Such a single underlying source viewed as an integral part of both a theoretical model and a corresponding clinical syndrome for DVD may result in a variety of motor, phonological, linguistic, or neurological signs or symptoms and in fact inconsistency among symptoms may be expected as typical. If this is the case, the argued distinction of whether DVD is a motor movement disorder or a linguistic disorder is irrelevant because the difficulty with organizing elements into larger and larger wholes would affect both movement and linguistic aspects of development. Taken further, DVD should not be considered a problem of elements per se whether they be articulatory postures, phonemes, morphemes, words, or sentences, but a problem of **bridging among the various elements** which constitute language performance. (pp. 119–120)

In other words, childhood apraxia affects the ability to plan a complex movement, especially the ability to combine movement units into a whole action. For example, at the executive level, one child may be able to produce individual consonant and vowel sounds, but not combine them into a fluent syllable. At the planning level, another child might be able to compose individual sentences about a story, but not organize them properly into a coherent narrative.

Hierarchical Levels of Phonology

A word is not merely a sequence of sounds glued together in a line. Parts of words, such as syllables, pattern as units. There are many specific theoretical models of the exact relationships among these units, but there is general agreement that the following units appear to be operative:

A **word**: is made up of one or more

feet: which are units of prosody or rhythm (as in poetry). Feet are made up of one or more

syllables: which also function as prosodic units. They are subject to certain language-specific limitations, such as the number of consonants that may occur in a sequence (consonant clusters) and whether syllable-final consonants are allowed. Syllables are made up of an

onset: the initial consonant or consonant cluster, if any, and a

rhyme: the remainder of the syllable. The rhyme includes a

nucleus: the part of the syllable that carries the pitch and loudness, usually a vowel or diphthong, and a

coda: the final consonant or cluster, if any.

Psycholinguistic studies have shown that even though the syllable is hard to define, most people are able to identify the number of syllables in a word. The rhyme of the syllable is the basis for rhyming in English and many other languages: for example, "cat," "bat," "hat," and "fat" all share the same rhyme: [æ t]. Onsets are the basis for **alliteration**, as in "many magenta marbles missed the mark." In slips of the tongue, onsets are usually repeated or switched around, leaving the rhymes intact, as in "a mig bess," "a mig mess," or "a big bess" for "a big mess." It is quite rare for a coda alone or a vowel alone to be repeated or switched in a slip of the tongue (as would be the case if someone said "a biss meg" or "a beg miss" for "a big mess").

Adult-Onset Versus Childhood Apraxia

Until recently, a major roadblock to understanding this disorder was the fact that far more information was available about **adult-onset apraxia of speech (AOS)**, a communication disorder that may result from a stroke or other neurological insult, than about CAS. Despite the common use of the term "apraxia," there are some critical differences between AOS and CAS. First, AOS is defined specifically as a purely motor speech articulation disorder. That is, if there are accompanying phonological, language, or other symptoms, these are categorized as a distinct disorder, such as Broca's aphasia (phonological and expressive language difficulties), Wernicke's aphasia (comprehension difficulties), or anomic aphasia (word-finding difficulties). Second, a person with AOS typically has a lifetime of overlearned, automatic speech to fall back on. Verbal routines (social niceties, songs, prayers, rhymes, expletives, counting, the alphabet, etc.) are usually still available to persons with AOS for communication purposes. Children with childhood apraxia have no such store of automatic speech, although verbal routines often prove easier for them to learn than more volitional speech acts. Indeed, many of them do not go through the normal prelinguistic babbling stages and therefore they lack even babble routines to rely upon. (See box on the importance of prelinguistic vocalizations.) The errors of children with CAS may be either inconsistent (as are adults') or consistent. Each child's level of consistency may also vary from sound to sound, word to word, sentence to sentence, day to day, and listener to listener; certain errors may occur only once, while others may appear to be quite permanent until suddenly they change completely. Therefore, inconsistency is not a reliable marker for apraxia in children.

DIFFERENTIAL DIAGNOSIS

It is important to differentiate between common symptoms of a disorder and specific symptoms that differentiate people with the disorder from people with other, similar, disorders. A major conundrum in this disorder area is the attempt to differentiate childhood apraxia from (other) phonological disorders, despite the fact that there is little agreement on exactly what the symptoms of CAS are. In some studies, certain characteristics (e.g., difficulties with **diadochokinesis** or **alternating repetitive motion tasks**) are taken to be hallmarks of the disorder and are used as selection criteria to identify subjects. These subjects are then studied to determine what other symptoms they share. Results of such studies identify symptoms that tend to co-occur with the researchers' subject selection criteria. Unfortunately, we do not know whether the co-occurring symptoms also occur in the absence of the selection criteria. As reported recently by McCabe, Rosenthal, and McLeod (1998), "many characteristics regarded as diagnostic for developmental dyspraxia occur in the general speech-impaired population" (p. 105). Perhaps the most potentially misleading studies are those in which a few children with a diagnosis of apraxia are compared to a group of normals, with the identified differences between the groups being taken as differentially diagnostic symptoms of apraxia (e.g., Marion, Sussman, & Marquardt, 1993; Marquardt, Sussman, Snow, & Jacks, 2002). Such symptoms may in fact be typical of children with phonological disorders in general, rather than specifically of children with apraxia.

In other studies, subjects are selected based upon a diagnosis of apraxia by a speech-language pathologist who is not associated with the study in any other way.

The Critical Role of Prelinguistic Vocalizations

Thelen (1981) proposes the following stages of motor control:

I. Uncoordinated movement: Individual limbs (or other body parts) move in apparently independent, random fashion.

II. **Rhythmic stereotypies**: Rhythmic movements of body parts produced repeatedly. The earliest examples include rhythmic sucking shortly after birth. This is followed by rhythmic kicking of both legs in unison, hand-banging of both arms in unison, whole-body rocking, and eventually canonical babbling (rhythmic "jaw-wagging"), which may initially be silent. According to Thelen, these rhythmic movement patterns provide practice in temporal patterning, leading to refinement of neuromotor control of the affected body parts.

III. Complex voluntary neuromotor control: Rhythmic kicking makes voluntary, purposeful kicking of one or both legs, either together or independently, possible; rocking "tunes up" the joints and muscles for coordinated crawling, and so forth. Similarly, rhythmic jaw movements ("bababa"; "dididi") facilitate the development of voluntary oral-motor control of the articulators.

Stoel-Gammon (1992), in a review of the literature, reports on the predictor value of prelinguistic vocalizations. Her review highlights the following relationships:

Amount of vocalization (at 3–6 months) correlates positively with:
- attention to reading (at 8 months)
- *Gesell Developmental Quotient* (at 9 months)
- rate of vocalization (at 13 months)
- *Bayley Verbal Scale* (at 11–15 months)
- vocabulary (at 27 months)

Percent use of **"true" consonants** (not glottals, not glides) in babble correlates positively with:
- age of child when his or her productive lexicon reaches 50 words
- phonological maturity (at 29, 36 months)
- *Preschool Language Scale* scores (at 6 years)

Use of idiosyncratic babble patterns at 9–16 months correlates with:
- expressive vocabulary (at 9–16 months)

Thus, the quality and quantity of an infant's prelinguistic vocalizations appear to serve as important precursors to meaningful speech. Children with CAS whose prelinguistic vocalizations may be lacking in quality, quantity, or both are therefore starting the speech game with a strike against them.

Such subject groups are far more heterogeneous, and the results are typically much more mixed. The most comprehensive study of this type was that described in Shriberg, Aram, and Kwiatkowski (1997a, b, c). In three different samples of children diagnosed with apraxia, they found that approximately 50% of the children in each sample exhibited **excess equal stress**, a pattern of monostressed (monoloud, monopitch) syllables and words that makes speech sound very robotic. The children in the study either exhibited this speech pattern frequently or very rarely; subjects appeared to be truly divided into two groups based upon this measure. This was the only aspect of the speech of the children with an apraxia diagnosis that reliably differentiated 50% of them from children with speech delay. (No one symptom could reliably differentiate the other 50% of the subjects with suspected apraxia from the speech-delayed group.) Shriberg et al. therefore propose excess equal stress as the best available criterion for differential diagnosis of CAS. However, the age ranges in this study were from 3 to almost 15 years of age. It is possible that, for at least some of the children, the excess equal stress pattern was a compensatory strategy for producing individual segments and syllables correctly at the expense of fluent prosody. This author has observed three children with apraxia who developed an excess equal stress pattern over time, possibly as a result of therapy focusing too heavily on segments, or as a result of preliteracy training in which the child was encouraged to count out syllables in a rhythmic, monotonic, monostress manner.

In an ongoing study, Velleman is administering a large body of tests to a group of children with moderate-severe phonological deficits. She is blind to the diagnoses of the individual children (i.e., whether anyone has ever labeled them "apraxic"). Her plan is to use cluster analysis to identify groups of symptoms that differentiate some of these children from others. Specifically, she hopes to determine whether a subgroup of her subjects will stand out from the others with respect to any of the characteristics commonly attributed to childhood apraxia of speech. This type of study is desperately needed to avoid the circularity that plagues many other studies of childhood apraxia.

The current "state of the art" is thus far from a tried-and-true recipe: no particular symptom in and of itself can be used to identify CAS. Rather, a thorough evaluation of the child's speech and language in a variety of dynamic communication contexts is required to identify a pattern of symptoms consistent with the disorder. Each child's particular profile is likely to change markedly as the child matures and benefits from intervention. If the diagnosis is appropriate, though, each new pattern of symptoms should continue to be consistent with a diagnosis of CAS.

INTERVENTION APPROACHES

The intervention approaches recommended by various practitioners and researchers are heavily dependent upon their view of the disorder and vice versa: the discovery of a remediation approach that works typically influences the discoverer's view of the nature of the disorder. Some approaches are quite motoric, dependent upon drill and focused upon the achievement of a hierarchy of articulatory gestures. Others incorporate linguistic components as well, with more emphasis on flexible, functional communication. The common thread among the vast majority of intervention approaches today is their emphasis upon the dynamic nature of speech. Rather than addressing the achievement of particular articulatory postures (i.e., the production of one consonant or vowel sound in isolation), most approaches emphasize the child's ability to transition smoothly from one posture to the next, in speech units at the level of the syllable and above.

PROGNOSIS

One classic feature of CAS has historically been lack of progress in therapy. Fortunately, this problem is apparently an artifact of therapy that was not ideally suited to the problem (i.e., therapy that did not address the dynamic nature of the disorder). Many children do progress slowly, in stair-step fashion, in which plateaus of little or no overt progress alternate with apparently sudden spurts of improvement. However, better intervention approaches, as well as earlier and more intense intervention, have made a significant difference in the prognosis of children with CAS. The disorder ranges from mild to severe (Hall, 1989; McCabe et al., 1998); in some cases, children who receive treatment early may appear to be symptom-free under normal, low-stress speaking circumstances by the time they reach first grade. Others require ongoing intervention well into their school years, and even into high school.

In some cases, more subtle linguistic difficulties or literacy-related difficulties may become apparent later in the middle school years, when academic tasks become more complex, sequential, and hierarchical. For example, some children with CAS are not identified as having difficulty with the auditory processing of complex sequences until fourth or fifth grade, when teachers' expectations of their students' ability to follow oral directions are much higher. This occurs frequently enough that some have hypothesized that it may be another, more subtle, symptom of childhood apraxia (K. Strand, personal communication). Similarly, a child who has no problem learning to read may begin to experience difficulty when she is expected to read to learn—that is, to acquire new concepts through reading rather than listening—especially when textbooks begin to include complex passages in which ideas or events are hierarchically related or are embedded within each other. In such cases, intervention may need to be reinstated for some period of time to address these more subtle deficits.

SECTION
2

SECTION

2

ASSESSMENT

··

Given the complexity of this disorder, and the ongoing debates about which symptoms are diagnostic, the diagnosis of childhood apraxia is complicated and challenging. In this section, various aspects of the assessment process will be discussed one by one, beginning with the child's history and background information. Those aspects of a speech-language assessment that are particularly diagnostic of childhood apraxia will be highlighted here.

PREASSESSMENT CONSIDERATIONS

- WHO? Children being assessed for phonological/phonetic delay/disorder with a question of childhood apraxia.
- WHAT? Red flags with special significance for a differential diagnosis of childhood apraxia.
- WHY? Not all symptoms need to be present, nor can any one symptom identify the disorder. Rather, a pattern of lack of coordination and planning skills and of difficulty with part-whole and whole-part combinations or sequences is diagnostic of childhood apraxia.
- LITERATURE RESOURCES: Aram (1984); Caruso & Strand (1999); Crary (1993); Hall, Jordan, & Robin (1993); Love (2000); Ripley, Daines, & Barrett (1997); Shriberg, Aram, & Kwiatkowski (1997a, b, c); E. Strand & McCauley (1999); Velleman & K. Strand (1994).

The characteristics listed here may be identified via case review, parent questionnaire, or preassessment interview. Some may also be observed directly by the clinician, and are therefore expanded upon later in this section.

Note: For any child who is not learning standard American English as a first language, special assessment procedures and techniques may be required. See Goldstein (2000) for further information.

Medical history
- **Soft neurological signs** (such as immature reflexes, mildly low muscle tone, and sensory **hypersensitivity** or **hyposensitivity**) may be noted or may have been noted in the past.

Family history of speech, language, hearing, or learning deficits
- In some cases apraxia does run in families.

Psychosocial history, including:
- High frustration levels of child and parent; resulting behavior management problems.
- Excessive shyness, especially in unfamiliar social settings.

History of feeding difficulties:
- Poor coordination of suck-swallow-breathe process, resulting in mild but frequent coughing/choking or spillage.
- Excessive drooling, especially when talking or engaged in other motor activities.

(If these symptoms are more than mild, an alternative or additional diagnosis of dysarthria should be considered.)

Speech oral-motor factors:
- Mandible is primary articulator.
  - Tongue does not move independently of jaw.
  - Stabilization of the mandible (e.g., speech-language pathologist's hand under child's chin) makes articulation more difficult.

- Groping or effort at initiation of speech may be evident.
- Difficulty organizing and sequencing segments in a variety of dynamic patterns.

Intelligibility:
- Big difference in intelligibility levels with closest family member (who has often learned to interpret the child's deviant **phonological patterns**, idiosyncratic gestures, and other communication patterns) versus other family members, less familiar interlocutors, and strangers.

Communicative means (age of onset; frequency of use):
- Prebabble vocalizations: few to no consonants; little vocal play; described as a quiet baby.
- Babble:
  —Little or no babbling, except for vowel-like vocalizations.
  —Limited differentiation of consonants and vowels in the babbling repertoire.
  —Little spontaneous imitation of syllables.
- **Jargon** ("speaking jibberish"; varied consonant and vowel patterns with appropriate intonation contours, but no apparent meaning): absent or very rare.
- Gesturing, leading parents to desired objects often heavily relied on.
- Family member cited as interpreter.
- Mime, sign: conventional or idiosyncratic (natural gesture system invented by child) or both.
- Words: signs/gestures, sound effects, and/or idiosyncratic words outnumber conventional intelligible words.
- Sentences: composed of combinations of oral words, signs, gestures.
  —Word or **morpheme** sequencing errors are present (e.g., "He's go" for "He goes"; "mowlawner" for "lawnmower").
  —Function words are omitted, mis-selected, or misplaced (e.g., "red big the ball" for "the big red ball").
- Receptive-expressive language gap, especially in children over 2 years of age.
- If child has had speech-language treatment in the past, progress may have been reported to be unusually slow.

Inconsistency:
- Child tends to produce a word once, then "lose" it.
- Child produces particular words in automatic contexts only; unable to reproduce or imitate on request.
- Accuracy of word production decreases when the length or phonetic difficulty of the utterance increases.
- Accuracy of word production varies with the conceptual or syntactic difficulty of the utterance; utterances that are shorter, less abstract, and grammatically simpler are also articulatorily clearer.
- Regression occurs
  —In unfamiliar contexts (situation, location, interlocutors, topic, etc.).
  —When task is altered or when a new task is introduced (e.g., child seems to have mastered [s], but then begins mispronouncing it again when [ʃ] is introduced).

Note: Since a child may exhibit the characteristics listed above **consistently**, the header "Inconsistency" is somewhat of a misnomer here. However, this term is typically used in the literature to describe these patterns of context-dependent change.

Play
- Age-appropriate, single-action **pretend play**, with delay in developing sequences of pretend play or nested pretend play episodes (actions with larger schemas).

Other sensory and motor factors
- Motor deficits
  —Muscle tone mildly low. (*Note:* Extreme tone differences usually accompany a neuromuscular disorder, such as cerebral palsy.)
  —Limb apraxia: Fine or gross motor-planning difficulties, especially for action sequences (hands, whole body).
- Sensory deficits
  —Mild to moderate sensory hypersensitivity, hyposensitivity, or both in different areas of the face and/or body.

Literacy
- Delayed rhyming skills
  —Difficulty with **segmentation** (of **compound words** into single words, multisyllabic words into syllables, monosyllabic words into onset-rhyme, monosyllabic words into segments, etc.).
  —Difficulty with **blending** (of words into compounds, syllables into multisyllabic words, onset-rhyme into monosyllabic words, segments into monosyllabic words).
  —Difficulty with whole-part, part-whole text analysis or composition (paragraphs, stories, etc.).

ORAL MECHANISM AND MOTOR SPEECH EXAMINATION

- WHO? Children being assessed for phonological/phonetic delay/disorder with a question of childhood apraxia.
- WHAT? Red flags with special significance for a differential diagnosis of childhood apraxia.
- WHY? Not all symptoms need to be present, nor can any single symptom identify the disorder. Rather, a pattern of lack of coordination and planning skills and of difficulty with part-whole and whole-part combinations or sequences is diagnostic of childhood apraxia.
- LITERATURE RESOURCES: Davis, Jakielski, & Marquardt (1998); Davis & Velleman (2000); Frick, Frick, Oetter, & Richter (1999); Hayden & Square (1999); Morris (1993); Oetter, Richter, & Frick (1995); E. Strand & McCauley (1999); Velleman & K. Strand (1994); Wells, Peppé, & Vance (1995).

Procedures for a complete oral mechanism/motor speech examination are suggested here. Some of the features listed below are used to confirm a diagnosis of dysarthria, rather than or in addition to a diagnosis of apraxia. Characteristics that are especially indicative of CAS are italicized.

Structure of the oral mechanism: Look for abnormalities or asymmetries of any of the following, as would normally be done in an oral mechanism examination.
- lips
- tongue
- hard palate
- soft palate
- nasopharynx

Function of the oral mechanism: (for structures listed earlier)
- Muscle tone: Children with apraxia may exhibit mildly low muscle tone, characterized by an open-mouth posture with the tongue held somewhat forward. However, this should not be used as a diagnostic characteristic, as it may co-occur with other disorders.
- Single movements (kiss, smile, protrude tongue, etc.): Note whether the child completes these on command or in imitation and how many trials are necessary.
- *Sequences of movements* (kiss, then smile; tongue out, to the side, then in, etc.): Look for effort, groping, mis-sequencing, irregular rhythm, **overshoot,** and **undershoot**.
- *More difficulty performing actions in imitation or pretend than functionally:* For example, compare the child's ability to lick a real lollipop or to actually brush his teeth versus his ability to pretend to do so or to imitate pretending to do so.
- *Difficulty transferring a learned motor skill to new contexts (poor stimulus generalization):* Look for indications that the child can perform a task in the environment in which he or she learned it, but not elsewhere.
- *Poor coordination of feeding, including:*
  —*Mild gagging/choking.*

—*Resistance to certain foods due to their texture, combinations of texture, taste, temperature.*

Note: Some children with apraxia may be hypersensitive, resulting in a preference for very smooth, bland, room-temperature foods. Others may be hyposensitive and need extra cues as to the location of the bolus in the mouth, such as extreme tastes (e.g., spicy or sour) or temperatures (hot or cold). In either case, foods that include more than one texture (such as spaghetti or cereal with milk) are often difficult for the child to process.

—**Stuffing**: *overfilling the mouth when eating, perhaps for increased sensory feed-back.*
—*Immature strategies for processing food in the mouth: sucking, squashing/swallowing,* **munching** *(chewing between front teeth), using fingers or utensils to move food to side for chewing.*
—Inadequate lip closure for retaining food in the mouth.
—*Apparent lack of awareness of food in the cheeks (pocketing) or on the lips, external cheeks, or chin; inability to clear the lips using the tongue.*

Note: If any of the feeding characteristics listed above is noted, a further feeding evaluation should be considered in order to investigate or rule out possible physiological or psychosocial causative factors.

Function of the oral mechanism for speech (as appropriate for age):
• Adequate oral air build-up for aspirated stops (crisp, not fricativelike): If deficient, this may be a sign of dysarthria or **velopharyngeal insufficiency**. Check for nasal air escape using a mirror beneath the nostrils.
• Adequate air build-up and precision of placement for fricatives (air is appropriately "squeezed").
• Adequate oral-nasal distinction: If deficient, this may be a sign of dysarthria or velopharyngeal insufficiency. Check for nasal air escape using a mirror beneath the nostrils.
• *Age-appropriate variations in rate, loudness, fluency, voice quality: Some children with apraxia have limited prosodic choices. For example, they may be able to speak loudly or softly, fast or slowly, but not in between. Others may demonstrate vocal harshness, especially hard glottal attack.*
• *Timing characteristics: The following phonological errors may be indicative of deficient motor planning with respect to timing:*
   —**Voicing errors:** [b] *for* /p/, [f] *for* /v/, *for example.*
   —**Affrication/deaffrication:** [tʃ] *for* /t/ *or vice versa, for example.*
   —**Epenthesis:** [bəlu] *for "blue,"* [ʃtu] *for "shoe," for example.*
• *Space characteristics*
   —*Shaping: Many children with apraxia have decreased awareness of the positions of their articulators (tongue, lips, etc.), which has a particularly striking effect on their production of less consonantal sounds, resulting in vowel deviations (vowels distorted or substituted for each other).*
   —*Precision*
      → undershoot: **frication of stops, centralization of vowels:** This may be indicative of dysarthria.

> → *overshoot:* **stopping of fricatives/other consonants; frication of liquids and glides; vowel deviations** *to extreme edges of* **vowel triangle** (i, a, u): *Due to reduced oral awareness, children with apraxia may overshoot in order to receive adequate sensory feedback.*
>
> → *placement errors:* **fronting** *(e.g., velars to alveolar, as in [ɛd] for "egg").* **backing** *(e.g., alveolar to velar, as in [gɪʃ] for "dish").*

Several additions and modifications to the usual oral-motor assessment protocol are often recommended specifically for apraxia. They include the following:

Syllable repetition (diadochokinesis; alternating motion rates)

- Rate each production on a scale from 0 to 5, depending on rhythmicity, accuracy, and the appropriateness of the rate at which it was produced. A good reproduction of the pattern rates 5. If rhythmicity, accuracy, and/or rate are compromised, subtract 1 point for each, and note the nature of the problem(s) as on Form 2–1. If the child is unable to perform the repetition at all, his or her score will be 0.
- Ask the child to repeat the same syllable (**reduplication,** e.g., [pʌpʌpʌpʌ]) and to repeat syllables while only varying consonants (alternating motion rates, e.g., [pʌtʌ], [pʌtʌkʌ]), as usual. In addition, ask the child to repeat syllables while only varying vowels (e.g., [tʌti], [tʌtitu]). Score as described above.

Suprasegmental Patterns

- Ask the child to vary his or her rate ("Let's say it really fast/slowly."), intonation patterns ("How would you ask your mom if you can have another cookie?") and **word stress** (*pre*sent as in "birthday present" verus pre*sent* as in "present an award"). This may be done in play, on request, or in imitation. Each item is rated based on the child's ability to perform the task appropriately.
- Vocal pitch, loudness, and quality are rated as appropriate or inappropriate, as they typically would be in an oral mechanism exam. **Nasal resonance** is evaluated by comparing the child's production of phrases that contain nasal consonants (e.g., "seventy-seven") versus those that do not (e.g., "eighty-eight").

Non-speech behaviors assessed are listed in Table 2-1.

One recent comprehensive (speech and non-speech) standardized oral-motor mechanism examination that is more child-friendly than many others is Hayden and Square's (1999) *Verbal Motor Production Assessment for Children* (VMPAC).

Table 2-1. Non-Speech Behaviors Form

Inaccuracies (including searching/groping behaviors), inappropriate rate, and/or number and types of cues provided are noted on the form below. Then, each item is rated based on the child's ability to perform the task appropriately.

5 = appropriate accuracy and rate without cue
4 = appropriate accuracy and rate with (one) auditory, visual, or tactile cue
3 = accuracy or rate inappropriate with maximum of one cue
2 = accuracy and rate inappropriate with maximum of one cue; or accuracy or rate inappropriate, with more than one type of cue required
1 = accuracy and rate inappropriate even with more than one type of cue
0 = unable to approximate even with cues

Action	Accuracy	Rate	Cue	Score
Stick out your tongue				
Blow				
Show teeth				
Pucker lips				
Touch nose with tip of tongue				
Bite lower lip				
Whistle				
Lick lips				
Clear throat				
Move tongue in and out				
Click teeth together once				
Smile				
Click tongue				
Cough				
Puff out cheeks				
Wiggle tongue side to side				
Pretend to kiss				
Alternately smile and pucker (kiss)				

Source: Adapted from K. Strand (1997).

COMMUNICATIVE MEANS

- **WHO?** Prelinguistic children being assessed for speech/language delay, especially those who are suspected of having childhood apraxia.
- **WHAT?** Assessment of prelinguistic vocal and gestural communication.
- **WHY?** The quality and quantity of prelinguistic vocalizations may be predictive of later language development (Stoel-Gammon, 1992); the quality of prelinguistic vocalizations may be indicative of childhood apraxia. Reliance on non-vocal communicative means may be indicative of childhood apraxia.
- **LITERATURE RESOURCES:** Bleile (1995); Fenson et al. (1993); Hedrick, Prather, & Tobin (1984); Kent & Bauer (1985); Olswang, Stoel-Gammon, Coggins, & Carpenter (1987); Proctor (1989); Reynell (1969); Stoel-Gammon (1989); Wetherby & Prizant (1993).

Vocal Communicative Means

Children with childhood apraxia tend to have reduced quantities of all of the following. In addition, the amount of variety in their vocalizations is often quite limited.

- Prebabble vocalizations: coo, gurgle; **vocal play** (e.g., screech, growl, click, raspberries, etc.).
- Babble: alternating consonants and vowels. If consonants are glottal stops, nasals, glides, or prolonged resonants/fricatives, this is considered to be **precanonical babble** (Oller, 1986). If "true" consonants (stops), then babble is **canonical**. Typically, precanonical and canonical babble are quite rhythmic.
- **Variegated babble**: Variety of consonants (including "true" consonants) and vowels, produced rhythmically.
- Jargon ("speaking gibberish," "telling stories"): Variety of consonants and vowels produced with sentencelike intonation contours and rhythm, but without any apparent meaning.

Table 2-2, the *Vocal Development Checklist* Form, is an adaptation of Proctor's (1989) *Developmental Vocal Assessment Protocol*. Vocal behaviors are listed according to the ages at which they are expected to occur. Each behavior judged to be within the child's vocal repertoire is to be indicated as "observed" by the examiner ("O") or "reported" by caregivers ("R"). In addition, behaviors that have been observed (by the examiner, caregivers, or both) rarely or only very recently may be indicated as "emerging" ("E").

Table 2-3 provides guidelines for using Stoel-Gammon's (1989) **Mean Babbling Level** measure. Each vocalization is rated as a level 1, level 2, or level 3 babble, based on the occurrence of "true" consonants within the vocalization, as defined in this table. Approximate age expectations for Mean Babbling Level (Stoel-Gammon, 1989) are given in Table 2-4. Table 2-5 provides one column for transcribing the child's vocalization, and another for indicating the corresponding babble level. The number of babbles at each level are added and multiplied by the numerical value of that level (e.g., number of level 3 babbles is multiplied by 3). The results are added and the sum is divided by the total number of vocalizations to yield the child's mean babbling level score. Alternatively, during a therapy or assessment session, the speech-language

Table 2-2. Vocal Development Checklist Form

Child's Name: _____ DOB: _____ Examiner: _____

Diagnosis: _____

Medical Factors: _____

Social Factors: _____

Assessment Dates: _____

Date	Age (CA or GA)	Vocal Level	Comments

O: Observed   R: Reported   E: Emerging (use with O or R)   C: Consonant   V: Vowel

Stage 1: Birth to Two Months

Rating	Behavior	Frequency/Transcription/Comments
O R E	Crying with sudden pitch shifts, extremely high pitch	
O R E	Fussing/discomfort	
O R E	Vegetative sounds (burps, feedings sounds)	
O R E	Neutral sounds (sighs, grunts)	
O R E	Ingressive vocalizations (vocalizing during inspiration)	
O R E	V-like sounds:	
	front V-like [i, ɪ, e, ɛ, æ]	
	mid V-like [ʌ ə]	
	back V-like [u, ʊ, o, ɔ, a]	
O R E	C-like sounds [k, h, ʔ, g, x, j, l, ɹ]	
O R E	Clicks, friction noises	
O R E	Trills (front, mid, back, uvular)	

(continues)

Table 2-2. (continued)

Stage 2: Two to Four Months

Rating	Behavior	Frequency/Transcription/Comments
O R E	Marked decrease in crying after 12 weeks	
O R E	Transition from primarily reflexive sounds	
O R E	Differential vocalizations related to state and context	
O R E	Vocalizes responsively+	
O R E	Mainly V-like sounds: [i, ɪ, e, ɛ, æ, ʌ, ə u, ʊ, ɔ, a]	
O R E	Occasional diphthongs	
O R E	Unrounded, often nasalized, central vowels	
O R E	Back V-like sounds frequent	
O R E	More Cs emerge [b, d, g, n, t, k, w, l, j, v, z, θ, h]	
O R E	Back/glottal C-like sounds [g, h, x, k, ʔ]	
O R E	More distinct friction sounds, trills	
O R E	Liquids (mainly trills)	
O R E	Voiced fricatives	
O R E	Nasals (syllabic nasals, nasalized vowels)	
O R E	Combinations of C with V: coo/goo [ʔə] or [gʌ]	
	single units (early stage 2)	
	in series/combination [əɣʊɣʊ] (mid- to late stage 2)	

+: Not listed in original DVAP.

(continues)

Table 2-2. (continued)

Stage 3: Four to Six/Seven Months

Rating	Behavior	Frequency/Transcription/Comments
O R E	Laughter emerges; voiced/voiceless alternations (haha)	
O R E	Vocal imitation (within own repertoire)+	
O R E	Pitch variations: rise, fall, fall-rise, rise-fall, rise-fall-rise	
O R E	Vocal play:	
	extreme pitch patterns	
	yell, squeal	
	low-pitched growl	
	variations in vocal quality	
	friction sounds: "raspberries," trills, smacks, snorts	
O R E	More varied Vs [i, ɪ, e, ɛ, æ, ʌ, ə, u, ʊ, o, ɔ, a]	
O R E	# of C-like sounds increases:	
	English-like: [m, n, b, d, g, ŋ, t, k, w, l, j, v, z, θ, h]	
	other: [ɣ, x, ʔ, Φ, ɲ, ʀ, ɯ, ç, ɕ]	
O R E	Marginal babble:	
	phonation interrupted by one C-like sound	
	series of C-like interruptions to phonation	

+: Not listed in original DVAP.

(continues)

Table 2-2. (continued)

Stage 4: Six/Seven to Ten Months

Rating	Behavior	Frequency/Transcription/Comments
O R E	Marked change: Vocalizations far more speechlike overall	
O R E	Consistent variation of intonation contours	
O R E	Varied, distinct Vs [i, ɪ, e, ɛ, æ, ʌ, ə, u, ʊ, o, ɔ, a, ɚ]	
O R E	Diphthongs increase [aɪ, oʊ, aʊ, eɪ]	
O R E	Cs increase, with fully stopped stops	
	English-like: [m, n, b, d, g, p, t, k, w, l, j, v, z, θ, h]	
	other: [ɣ, x, ʔ, Φ, ɲ, ʀ, ɯ, ç, ɕ, ʂ, ʍ, ʒ, ð]	
O R E	Series of canonical babble syllables	
	reduplicated, rhythmic (babababa)	
	smooth transitions between C and V; between syllables	
	produced in turn-taking routines with caregiver+	
	syllabic imitation (within own repertoire)+	
	variegated: change in V or C within sequence*	
	jargon: speechlike intonation contour*	
O R E	Parents identify "1st word" (e.g., "mama") (10 ms.)*	

+: Not listed in original DVAP.
*: May not emerge until next stage.

(continues)

Table 2-2. (continued)

Stage 5: Ten to Twelve Months

Rating	Behavior	Frequency/Transcription/Comments
O R E	Sentencelike prosodic contours:	
	falling (as in declaratives)	
	steadily rising (as in Y/N questions)	
	sharp rise (as in imperatives)	
O R E	Increasingly varied, more speechlike vocalizations:	
	variegated babble: change in V or C within sequence	
	speechlike intonation contour	
	syllables not restricted to CV*	
	more fricative and "other" Cs in jargon+	
O R E	Meaningful vocal communication:	
	phonetically consistent forms (e.g., squeal at cat)+	
	approximations of single words	
	approximations of phrases (e.g., "I love you")+*	
	"fills in the blanks" in verbal routines (e.g., book)+*	

+: Not listed in original DVAP.
*: May not emerge until next stage.
Source: Adapted from Proctor (1989).

Table 2-3. Mean Babbling Level

Babble Level	Description	Examples
1	No true consonants	ʔəʔ, ijɛ, wɑʊwɑʊwɑʊ
2	One true C (may be repeated)	ɑbɑp, didɑdidɑ
3	At least two different true Cs	mɑdi, ɑbinəbinə, gɪp

Source: Adapted from Stoel-Gammon (1989).

pathologist may choose simply to keep a count of numbers of babbles in each category (levels 1, 2, 3), thereby deriving the child's mean babble level without transcribing each vocalization. *Note:* Mean Babbling Level is typically lower in first words than in variegated babble and jargon; thus, it may decrease when the child begins to produce adult-based words.

Definitions:

"True" consonants are:

- **supraglottal** (i.e., not [h], not [ʔ])
- not glides (not [w] or [j])

"Different" consonants:

- differ from each other in place or manner of articulation or both (based on broad transcription).
- may or may not differ from each other in voicing. (Voicing is not taken into account when calculating MBL, as children at this age or level frequently produce segments with intermediate voicing, and transcription of their voicing has been found to be quite unreliable.)

Table 2-4. Approximate Age Expectations for Mean Babbling Level

Age (in months)	# of Subjects	Average MBL
9	32	1.33
12	32	1.50
15	24	1.58
18	8	1.65

Source: Adapted from Stoel-Gammon (1989; Table 1, p. 214).

Non-Vocal Communicative Means

It is not unusual for children with childhood apraxia to rely on gesture, leading, or mime to get their points across. Some may be quite creative, even using their own idiosyncratic signs to form sentences or even stories. Others may combine oral words (or word attempts) with gestures or signs.

Thus, use of any of the following should be documented:

1. Single natural gesture (e.g., hands raised for "pick me up").
2. Combination of natural gestures (e.g., point to cabinet, then raise hands for "pick me up to see in the cabinet").

3. Combination of natural gesture plus word attempt (e.g., "daddy" plus pat floor to indicate that father should sit down there).
4. Idiosyncratic sign, that is, gestures that take on specific meanings for the child (e.g., twist hand to request being twirled around by adult).
5. Conventional signs (e.g., fingertips tapped together to request "more").
6. Combinations of the above.

Table 2-6 can be used to document **communicative intents** (the meaning that the child is trying to convey) and **communicative means** (the way that he or she tries to convey it). For each communicative intent observed, the speech-language pathologist should note on the form whether the child conveyed this meaning vocally (with a babble, a screech, an oral word, etc.) or non-vocally (with a gesture, facial expression, body movement, sign, etc.).

Table 2-5. Mean Babbling Level Form

Vocalization (Transcription)	Babble Level

Note: Ideally, at least 50 vocalizations should be used.

# of vocalizations at level 1: _____ × 1 = _____

# of vocalizations at level 2: _____ × 2 = _____

# of vocalizations at level 3: _____ × 3 = _____

Total # of vocalizations: _____

Sum _____

Sum ÷ total # of vocalizations = _____ = MBL

Table 2-6. Communicative Intents and Communicative Means Form

Communicative Intent	Vocal Means	Non-Vocal Means
Greet		
Call		
Request (action)		
Request (answer)		
Protest		
Label		
Repeat or imitate		
Initiate activity or dialogue		
Take turns		
Maintain topic		
Describe events		
Role-play		

PHONOLOGICAL ASSESSMENT: OVERVIEW

- WHO? Children being assessed for phonological/phonetic delay/disorder with a question of childhood apraxia.
- WHAT? Red flags with special significance for a differential diagnosis of childhood apraxia.
- WHY? Not all symptoms need to be present, nor can one single symptom alone identify the disorder. Rather, a pattern of lack of coordination and planning skills and of difficulty with part-whole and whole-part combinations or sequences is diagnostic of childhood apraxia.
- LITERATURE RESOURCES: Davis, Jakielski, & Marquardt (1998); Davis & MacNeilage (1995); Davis & Velleman (2000); E. Strand & McCauley (1999); Velleman (1994, 1998); Velleman & K. Strand (1994).

Clinical Note:
Particularly with a child under 8 years of age, it is important to consider that two issues coexist:

1. A child's developing phonological system, which may include appropriately or inappropriately immature phonological patterns or processes.
2. A child's attempts to compensate for phonetic performance difficulties, which may result in unusual phonological patterns.

Areas for Assessment

The ideal assessment should include the areas listed below.

Note: Those areas that are especially indicative of apraxia are in italics. Each area will be explained in more depth in the following pages.

Phonotactics (syllable and word shapes)
- *Relatively poor repertoire of syllable and word shapes* (e.g., reduplicated CVCV only).
- *Developmentally unexpected syllable/word shape repertoire* (e.g., VC syllables predominate).
- *Reduced flexibility:*
   —*limited C + V combinations (certain Cs co-occur with certain Vs only).*
   —*certain Cs occur in certain positions only (e.g., final).*
- *High number of sequencing errors* (e.g., **migration, metathesis**).

Phonetic repertoire (consonants and vowels)
- *Limited repertoires of consonants and/or vowels.*
- *Developmentally unexpected phonetic repertoires* (e.g., child produces [k] but not [d], or [aʊ] but not [i]).
- Age-inappropriate level of phonemic contrast: contrastive phones not used in contrastive manner (e.g., Cs are always voiced in initial position, voiceless in final position, eliminating the possibility of a voice contrast).

Patterns **(phonological processes** or **constraints)**
- Age-appropriateness of patterns/processes (immature processes are not present).
- *Timing-related processes*: *voicing*/**devoicing**, *affrication/deaffrrication, epenthesis.*
- Space-related processes:
  - —*Shaping: vowel deviations*
  - —Precision:
    - → Undershoot (frication, centralization)
    - → *Overshoot*: : *stopping, frication of liquids or glides, vowel deviations to extreme edges of vowel triangle ([i, a, u])*
    - → Placement errors (fronting, backing)

Prosody
- *Age-inappropriate word stress,* **phrase stress,** *or* **sentence stress** *patterns.*
- *Age-inappropriate loudness or pitch patterns.*

Communicative effectiveness
- Intelligibility
- Number of **homonym**s (words that sound the same, but have different meanings)
- Level of consistency

PHONOLOGICAL ASSESSMENT: PHONOTACTIC REPERTOIRE

- WHO? Children being assessed for phonological/phonetic delay/disorder with a question of childhood apraxia.
- WHAT? Focus on phonotactics (word and syllable shapes).
- WHY? This is often an area of particular difficulty for children with apraxia.
- LITERATURE RESOURCES: Grunwell (1985); Hodson (1986); Ingram (1981); Shriberg & Kwiatkowski (1980); Bankson & Bernthal (1990); Kirkpatrick, Stohr, & Kimbrough (1990); Velleman & K. Strand (1994); Velleman (1998).

Areas for Assessment

Syllable shapes

Children with apraxia may have particular difficulty producing certain syllable shapes, such as those that include a final consonant or a cluster.

Check for the occurrence of the syllable shapes shown in Table 2-7.

Word shapes and stress patterns

Children with apraxia may have particular difficulty producing two (or more) different segments or syllables within the same word or with certain stress patterns within a word. Check for the occurrence of the word shapes and stress patterns shown in Table 2-8.

Table 2-7. Syllable Shapes by Approximate Age

Syllable Shapes	Example	Expected by Age[a] (in months)
C alone (incomplete syllable)	mmm	infancy; represents a *small* proportion of vocalizations beyond 8–10 months;
V alone (incomplete syllable)	aaahhh	frequency decreases from 8–12 months on
CV	go	12
CVC:		
C harmony (same)	pup	18–24
Different Cs	dog	24–30
CCV	play	36
CCVC	clam	36
VCC	ant	36–48
CVCC	paint	36–48
CCVCC, CCCVC, etc.		48 and later

Source: Compiled from Grunwell (1985), Chin & Dinnsen (1992), Smit et al. (1990), and Stoel-Gammon (1987).
[a]Ages are *approximate.*

Table 2-8. Word Shapes/Stress Patterns by Approximate Age of Appearance

Word Shapes	Examples	Age (in months)
One syllable	ma, pop	8–12
Two syllables:		
same Cs	daddy	8–12
different Cs	bottle	12–18
SW stress	*daddy*	8–12
WS stress	*giraffe*	36
Three syllables:		
SWS stress	*crocodile*	36
WSW stress	ban*a*na	36–42
Longer words:		
initial weak syllable	re*frige*rator	48 or later
initial strong syllable	*pedia*trician	48 or later

S: strong (stressed) syllable.
W: weak (unstressed) syllable.

Word shape error patterns

Check for the occurrence of the word shape error patterns listed below. Patterns that persist beyond the ages given below, especially if they occur very frequently, may be indicative of childhood apraxia.

Up to 18 Months

Reduplication, for example, "bottle" pronounced as [bɑbɑ].

Note: May persist in particular words, especially if parents imitate the form.

Consonants and vowels within syllables agree in place of articulation.
- Tongue-tip consonants co-occur only with tongue-tip vowels, for example, "daddy" as [dɪdɪ].
- Back consonants co-occur only with back vowels, for example, "giggle" as [gugu].
- Lip consonants co-occur only with open-jaw vowels, for example, "mommy" as [mɑmɑ].

Up to 30 Months

Consonant harmony, for example, "doggie" produced as [dɔdɪ].

Metathesis/migration: Consonants change places, for example, "Grampa" as [pɑgɑ] or "bug" as [gʌb]

Note: Some changes (such as [dɛks] for "desk") may be correct in some dialects.
Metathesis may persist longer in longer words, for example, "spaghetti" as [gəspɛɾi].

Syllable sequencing errors: whole syllables or words in a compound change places, for example, "doghouse" for "housedog."

PHONOLOGICAL ASSESSMENT: PHONETIC REPERTOIRE

- WHO? Children being assessed for phonological/phonetic delay/disorder with a question of childhood apraxia.
- WHAT? Focus on phonetics: individual sounds.
- WHY? This is an area of difficulty for most children with any type of phonological/phonetic delay/disorder.
- LITERATURE RESOURCES: Bleile (1995); Grunwell (1985); Hodson (1986); Ingram (1981); Shriberg & Kwiatkowski (1980); Bankson & Bernthal (1990); Kirkpatrick, Stohr, & Kimbrough (1990); Velleman & K. Strand (1994); Velleman (1998).

Using a speech sample, naming, or imitation task, detemine whether the child produces consonants:
- at a variety of places of articulation. These typically emerge in the following order:
  —Labial, alveolar
  —Labiodental, velar
  —Interdental, palatal
- using a variety of manners of articulation. These typically emerge in the following order:
  —Stop, glide, nasal
  —Fricative
  —Liquid, affricate

Table 2-9 shows Stoel-Gammon's (1987) findings on early consonantal repertoires. Table 2-10 shows the phonetic characteristics of American English consonants.

Table 2-11 can be used to document a particular child's consonant inventory. One copy of this form may be filled out for each word position in which the child produces consonants: initial, medial, and/or final. Consonants that are produced at least three times per 100 words in that word position should be documented. Those that are produced fewer than three times per 100 words, considered to be emerging, are also recorded, but in parentheses to indicate their reduced frequency of occurrence.

Determine, using a speech sample or a naming or imitation task, whether the child produces vowels:
- That differ with respect to the height of the tongue in the oral cavity (e.g., [i] versus [ɑ]).
- That differ with respect to the front-back placement of the tongue in the oral cavity (e.g., [i] versus [u]).

Table 2-9. Early Consonantal Repertoires

Age (in months)	# Subjects	Phone Classes
15	7	voiced stop, h
18	19	voiced stop, nasal, glide w, h
21	32	voiced stop, nasal, glide w, h
24	33	voiced and voiceless stop, nasal, glide, fricative

Source: Adapted from Stoel-Gammon (1987).

Table 2-10. Phonetic Characteristics of American English Consonants

Place → Manner ↓	Labial	Interdental	Alveolar	Palatal	Velar	Glottal
Stop *voiced* *voiceless*	b p		d t		g k	?
Nasal	m		n		ŋ	
Glide	w			j		
Fricative *voiced* *voiceless*	v f	ð θ	z s	ʒ ʃ		
Affricate *voiced* *voiceless*				dʒ tʃ		
Liquid			l	ɹ		

Table 2-11. Consonant Inventory Form

Word Position (circle one):　　Initial　　Medial　　Final　　All

Place → Manner ↓	Labial	Interdental	Alveolar	Palatal	Velar	Glottal
Stop *voiced* *voiceless*						
Nasal						
Glide						
Fricative *voiced* *voiceless*						
Affricate *voiced* *voiceless*						
Liquid						

At least [i, ɑ, u] should be present for young or severely involved children.

Table 2-12 shows the phonetic characteristics of American English vowels. Table 2-13 provides space for noting the vowels that are present in a given child's inventory. Again, include the vowels that are produced at least three times per 100 words. Vowels that are produced, but less frequently, are also recorded, in parentheses.

Because children with mild to moderate apraxia may have better than expected phonetic inventories, it is important to compare phonetic and phonotactic repertoires. It is common for children with apraxia to exhibit a **chronological mismatch** (Grunwell, 1985); that is, there may be other aspects of phonology that are significantly more delayed than the child's phonetic repertoire alone would indicate. Table 2-14 facilitates the comparison of the child's phonetic and phonotactic repertoires. Check the phonotactic patterns that the child exhibits. Then determine an approximate age level by identifying the "Phonotactic Patterns" box that most closely matches the child's productions. On the right side of the form, circle consonants that occur at least three times per 100 words. Determine an approximate age level by identifying the "Phonetic Repertoire" box that most closely matches the child's productions. If the age level of the child's phonotactic pattern does not match the age level of his or her phonetic repertoire, this indicates a chronological mismatch.

Table 2-12. Phonetic Characteristics of American English Vowels

Front-Back → Height ↓	Front	Central	Back
High *tense* *lax*	i ɪ		u ʊ
Mid *tense* *lax*	e ɛ		o ɔ
Low	æ	ʌ, ə	ɑ

Table 2-13. Vowel Inventory Form

Front-Back → Height ↓	Front	Central	Back
High *tense* *lax*			
Mid *tense* *lax*			
Low			

Table 2-14. Phonetic Versus Phonotactic Repertoire Form

KEY: C: consonant   ( ), e: emerging
        V: vowel
        CC: consonant cluster (generic)
        CCC: cluster with three or more Cs

Age	Phonotactic Patterns (check if present)	Phonetic Repertoire (circle if occurs three times)

1;6–2;0	___initial C
	___two-syllable words with:
	   ___reduplication
	   ___C harmony
	   ___V harmony
	   ___syllable reduction from iambics
	   ___CC reduction
	   ___final C deletion
		m n
		b p
		w
		
		                              h

2;0–2;6	___initial C
	___two-syllable with no harmony
	   or reduplication
	___syllable reduction from iambic words
	___CC reduction
	___final C deletion *or* final C harmony
		m n ŋ
		b p d t g k
		w
		
		                              h

2;6–3;0	___initial C ___two-syllable words with no harmony or reduplication ___syllable reduction from iambic words ___CC reduction ___final C without C harmony	m n ŋ b p d t g k w j f h

3;0–3;6	___initial C
	___two-syllable words with no
	   harmony or reduplication
	___syllable reduction from iambic
	   words longer than two syllables
	___some stop + glide initial CC
	___medial and final CC reduction
	___final C without C harmony
		m n ŋ
		b p d t g k
		w j
		v f s ʃ h
		                 tʃ
		        l (ɹ)

3;6–4;6	___initial C
	___two to three-syllable words with
	   no harmony, reduplication, or
	   reduction
	___stop + glide initial CC
	___some medial and final CC
	___final C without C harmony
		m n ŋ
		b p d t g k
		w j
		v f s ʃ h
		              dʒ tʃ
		        l (ɹ)

Table 2-14. (*continued*)

Age	Phonotactic Patterns (check if present)	Phonetic Repertoire (circle if occurs three times)
4;6–7;0	____initial C ____two to three-syllable words with no harmony, reduplication, or reduction ____four-+-syllable words (initially with harmony, reduplication, or reduction) ____all CC except θɹ- ____final C without C harmony	m n ŋ b p d t g k ʔ w j v f ð θ z s (ʒ) ʃ h dʒ tʃ l ɹ
7;0–9;0	____initial C ____multisyllabic words with no harmony, reduplication, or reduction ____all CC including θɹ-, all positions ____CCC in all positions ____final C without C harmony	m n ŋ b p d t g k ʔ w j v f ð θ z s (ʒ) ʃ h dʒ tʃ l ɹ

Sources: Compiled from Grunwell (1985), Bleile (1995), and Velleman (1998).

PHONOLOGICAL ASSESSMENT: PATTERNS/PROCESSES

- WHO? Children being assessed for phonological/phonetic delay/disorder with a question of childhood apraxia.
- WHAT? Focus on error patterns.
- WHY? Certain error patterns, especially those that relate to timing, space, or sequencing, are common among children with apraxia.
- LITERATURE RESOURCES: Bankson & Bernthal (1990); Grunwell (1985); Hodson (1986); Ingram (1981); Khan & Lewis (1986); Shriberg (1986); Shriberg & Kwiatkowski (1980); Stoel-Gammon, Stone-Goldman, & Glaspey (2002); Velleman (1998); Weiner (1979).

Many children who do not have apraxia exhibit some of the phonological processes to be discussed below. Apraxia is indicated only if several error patterns are noted. Those that are particularly indicative of apraxia, especially when they are identified in children over age 3, include reduplication, **harmony, initial consonant deletion,** migration/metathesis, epenthesis, vowel deviations, and **unstressed syllable deletion/augmentation**. These patterns can be grouped according to the fundamental difficulty that underlies each one: timing, articulatory space, and sequencing (whole-word planning). These groups are listed, with examples of the relevant processes, below.

Timing error patterns:
- Voicing errors (e.g., [dɔk] for "dog"; [bɑp] for "pop")
- Affrication (e.g., [tʃɑk] for "sock")
- Deaffrication (e.g., [ʃiz] or [tiz] for "cheese")
- **Nasalization** (e.g., [mʌŋk] for "book")
- **Denasalization** (e.g., [bæk] for "bank")
- **Consonant cluster coalescence** (e.g., [fɪŋ] for "swing")

Space/accuracy error patterns:
- Fronting (e.g., [tʊti] for "cookie")
- Backing (e.g., [ku] for "two")
- Vowel deviations (e.g., [snæk] for "snake")

Whole-word error patterns:
- Reduplication (e.g., [bɛbɛ] for "Betsy")
- Consonant harmony (e.g., [gɔgi] or [dɔdi] for "doggie")
- Migration: one sound is moved (e.g., [nos] for "snow")
- Metathesis: two sounds change places (e.g., [gʌb] for "bug")
- Epenthesis: addition of sounds or syllables (e.g., [bʌnənænə] for "banana," [æpsəl] for "apple")
- Initial consonant deletion (e.g., [ɪnɚ] for "dinner")
- Omissions of weak (unstressed) syllables (e.g., [nænə] for "banana")
- Augmentation of weak syllables (e.g., [bænænə] for "banana")

Use Table 2-15 to record phonological processes. Note errors made on the line following each process.

Table 2-15. Phonological Processes Common in Childhood Apraxia Form

A. Timing

Voicing errors (e.g., [dɔk] for "dog"; [bɑp] for "pop")

Affrication (e.g., [tʃɑk] for "sock")

Deaffrication (e.g., [ʃiz] or [tiz] for "cheese")

Nasalization (e.g., [mʌŋk] for "book")

Denasalization (e.g., [bæk] for "bank")

Consonant cluster coalescence (e.g., [fɪŋ] for "swing")

B. Space/Accuracy

Fronting (e.g., [tʊti] for "cookie")

Backing (e.g., [ku] for "two")

Vowel deviations (e.g., [snæk] for "snake")

C. Sequencing/whole-word processing

Reduplication (e.g., [bɛbɛ] for "Betsy")

Consonant harmony (e.g., [gɔgi] or [dɔdi] for "doggie")

Migration: one sound is moved (e.g., [nos] for "snow")

Metathesis: two sounds change places (e.g., [gʌb] for "bug")

Epenthesis of sounds or syllables (e.g., [bʌnənænə] for "banana", [æpsəl] for "apple")

Initial consonant deletion (e.g., [ɪnɚ] for "dinner")

Omissions of weak (unstressed) syllables (e.g., [nænə] for "banana")

Augmentation of weak syllables (e.g., [bænænə] for "banana")

PHONOLOGICAL ASSESSMENT: PROSODY

- WHO? Children being assessed for phonological/phonetic delay/disorder with a question of childhood apraxia.
- WHAT? Focus on prosody.
- WHY? This is often an area of particular difficulty for children with apraxia.
- LITERATURE RESOURCES: Crystal (1981); Gerken (1991, 1994a, b); Gerken & McIntosh (1993); Hargrove & McGarr (1994); Kehoe (1995, 1997); Kehoe & Stoel-Gammon (1997b); Shriberg, Aram, & Kwiatkowski (1997a, b, c); Velleman & Shriberg (1999); Wells, Peppe & Goulandris (2001); Wells & Peppe (2001).

Areas for Assessment

Note: Areas that may raise concerns about possible apraxia are in italics.

Rate, volume, nasality
- *Inappropriate loudness patterns or* **monoloudness** (debated in the apraxia literature).
- *Inappropriate or inconsistent hypernasality/hyponasality* (debated in the apraxia literature).

Multisyllabic words mis-stressed or **monostressed** (Velleman & Shriberg, 1999).

Weak syllables omitted from multisyllabic words beyond age 6 (Velleman & Shriberg, 1999).

Sentences mis-stressed or monostressed (Shriberg, Aram, & Kwiatkowski, 1997c).

Inappropriate pitch patterns or **monopitch** (debated in the apraxia literature).

TYPICAL ERRORS UP TO AGE 3 (AND BEYOND): OMIT WEAK (UNSTRESSED) SYLLABLES

In initial position
Example: "banana" pronounced as [nænə]

In medial position
Example: "dinosaur" pronounced as [dɑɪsoɚ]

Sometimes a whole strong + weak pair of syllables (a foot) in initial position may even be omitted in a long word, if the strongest syllable comes near the end of the word:
Example: "hippopotamus" pronounced as [pɑ́rəmʌs]

In certain words, these same patterns continue into normal adult casual speech:
Examples:
- "parade" is pronounced as [pɹeɪd]
- "library" is pronounced as [lɑɪbɹi]
- "sonata" is pronounced as [snɑrə]
- In Britain, "medicine" is pronounced as [mɛdsɪn]

However, persistence of typical but non-adult errors beyond age 3 may indicate a speech delay; persistence beyond age 6 may be indicative of childhood apraxia (Velleman & Shriberg, 1999).

Atypical Errors:
(possibly indicative of childhood apraxia; Velleman & Shriberg, 1999)

Omit stressed syllables (only) from any position:
Example: "baby" pronounced as [bi]

Overstress weak syllables in a word, yielding an excess equal stress pattern
Example: "spaghetti" pronounced as [spágéti]

Overstress weak words in a sentence, yielding an excess equal stress pattern. For example, every word in the sentence is pronounced as stressed so no contrast between stressed and unstressed words can be identified (Shriberg, Aram, & Kwiatkowski, 1997c).

A new prosody test, currently in the norming stage in Britain, assesses children's receptive and expressive prosody skills, with respect to both function (e.g., understanding that a rise in pitch indicates a question) and form (e.g., identifying when a pitch rise occurs). Developed by Peppé and Wells, it is called *Profiling Elements of Prosodic Systems.*

PHONOLOGICAL ASSESSMENT: COMMUNICATIVE EFFECTIVENESS

- WHO? Children being assessed for phonological/phonetic delay/disorder with a question of childhood apraxia.
- WHAT? Focus on communicative effectiveness/intelligibility.
- WHY? The purpose of phonology is to get one's point across. Communicative effectiveness is an important indicator of severity from a functional point of view.
- LITERATURE RESOURCES: Bleile (1995); Gordon-Brannan (1994); Grunwell (1985); Ingram (1981); Kent (1992); Shriberg & Kwiatkowski (1983); Velleman (1994).

If a child produces many homonyms or produces the same word very inconsistently (in a different way each time), then he or she will be difficult to understand and will not communicate effectively.

Homonyms

A large number of homonyms reduces the child's communicative effectiveness. If too many words sound the same, the listener cannot guess the intended meaning. Use Table 2-16 to document homonyms. List the phonetic form of the homonym on the left, and its meanings in the child's vocabulary on the right. It is normal for children of any age to have some homonyms; adults certainly do (e.g., "do, dew, due"). Homonyms are especially prevalent under the age of 24 to 28 months. By the time the child is 3 years of age, the majority of his or her words (i.e., 80% or more) should be distinct (i.e., not homonyms).

Inconsistency

Although consistency is not a reliable measure for differential diagnosis of CAS, it is strongly related to intelligibility. A large degree of inconsistency reduces the child's communicative effectiveness. If the child's word productions are very inconsistent, the listener cannot learn to differentiate individual words; it's not possible to learn a pattern if there is none!

One way to document inconsistency is given in Table 2-17. List the meaning on the left, and the varying phonetic forms that the child uses to express that meaning on the right.

Another measure of consistency is the Consistency Index (Tyler, 2002). For this measure, the number of different substitutes (including substitution of nothing, i.e., deletion) a child uses for each targeted phoneme is calculated. These numbers can then be summed and divided by the number of phonemes targeted (attempted) to derive a Consistency Average, as shown in Table 2-18.

Table 2-16. Homonyms Form

List phonetic forms that the child uses with two or more meanings.

Phonetic Form	Meanings
EX: [bɑ]	ball, balloon, bye

Table 2-17. Inconsistency Form

List words that the child produces using more than one different phonetic form.

Meaning   **Phonetic Forms**

EX: balloon   [bɑ, bʊ, bɑbu, nu, un]

Table 2-18. Consistency Average Form

Target Phoneme	Substitutions (including ∅)			Total # of Substitutions for That Phoneme*
	Initial Substitutions	*Medial Substitutions*	*Final Substitutions*	

Total number of substitutions ÷ total number of phonemes attempted = Consistency Average.

The smaller the Consistency Average, the more consistent the child's speech patterns. For example, a child who averages only one substitution per phoneme (Consistency Average = 1.0) is very consistent; a child who averages three substitutions per phoneme (Consistency Average = 3.0) is not.

*Note: Substitutions that occur in multiple word positions only count once. For example, if a child substitutes [t] for /k/ in initial, medial, and final positions, only one substitution is counted in the far right column, because that one substitution is consistent across all word positions. Substitutions (or omissions) that occur within consonant clusters are counted in the same manner as singleton consonants.

LANGUAGE CHARACTERISTICS

- WHO? Children being assessed for combined language and phonological/phonetic delay/disorder with a question of childhood apraxia.
- WHAT? Focus on error patterns that are typical of the language of children with apraxia.
- WHY? Certain error patterns, especially those that relate to sequencing, are common among children with apraxia.
- LITERATURE RESOURCES: Bankson (1990); Carrow (1974); Carrow-Woolfolk (1999); Crystal, Fletcher, & Garman (1976); Bzoch & League (1991); Dunn & Dunn (1997); Gardner (2000a); German (2000); Goldsworthy (1982); Hresko, Reid, & Hammill (1999); Lee (1974); Long & Fey (1993); Miller & Chapman (1995); Retherford (1993); Semel, Wiig, & Secord (1992, 1995); Shipley & McAfee (1992); Shulman (1986); Stickler (1987); Tyack & Gottsleben (1974); Wallace & Hammill (1997); Weiss (2001); Zachman et al. (1978); Zimmerman, Steiner, & Pond (1992).

Areas for Assessment That May Be Indicative of Apraxia

Receptive-expressive language gap: Receptive language is significantly better than expressive language. Typically, receptive language is within normal limits. If receptive language is not within normal limits, then some other diagnosis (such as specific language disorder, developmental delay, central auditory processing disorder, etc.) may be primary, with CAS as a secondary or inappropriate diagnosis. Use receptive and expressive language test scores to determine whether the child demonstrates a chronological mismatch with respect to grammar or vocabulary. If the child's expressive language appears to be delayed or formal testing is inconclusive (due to bidialectism, bilingualism, attention deficits, or other factors), more naturalistic means, such as Mean Length of Utterance, should be used to gather further details about the child's expressive language. (See Weiss, 2001, for further discussion of naturalistic procedures for analyzing children's language samples.)

Mean Length of Utterance (MLU): Collect a language sample to determine the child's MLU (as described by e.g., Shipley & McAfee, 1992; Stickler, 1987; Weiss 2001). For children with poor intelligibility, transcription and analysis can be facilitated if the context is controlled (e.g., with a certain set of toys). It is also helpful to have an adult who is familiar with the child present to respond in such a way as to make the child's meaning clear (e.g., "I see. The doggie is eating the fish."). MLU is often low for chronological/mental age in children with apraxia, due to:
- omission of function words.
- combinations of gesture + word used to achieve multiword utterances.
- longer utterances that are unintelligible and therefore not included in MLU.

Word-sequencing errors: Search the language sample for sentences in which words are not in the correct grammatical order.
- free morphemes out of order (e.g., "Beep pick-up trucks not" = "Pick-up trucks don't beep").
- misplaced bound morphemes (e.g., "A rock don't floats" = "A rock doesn't float").

Early grammatical milestones are summarized in Table 2-19.

Word-finding difficulties: Children with phonological disorders of any sort may exhibit word-finding difficulties of three types:

- Apparent semantic substitutions: Often, this is a strategy that the child uses to avoid producing phonologically difficult words. For example, the child might say "Saint Nick" instead of "Santa Claus" and "lobster" instead of "crab" because he is aware of his own difficulty in pronouncing initial [k] + liquid clusters. In these cases, there is a consistent relationship between the substitutions and the target words:
    - —the targets contain sounds or sequences that the child is aware are difficult for him.
    - —the substitution words are easier for that particular child to pronounce.
- Actual phonemic substitutions: Far less often, a child with a phonological disorder may make retrieval errors in which a phonetically similar word is retrieved instead of the target (e.g., "banister" for "canister"). These substitution words are typically
    - —not semantically related to the targets.
    - —not phonologically easier than the targets.
- Actual semantic substitutions: Children with both a phonological and a semantic language disorder (or just a semantic disorder) may exhibit substitutions of related words for non-phonological reasons, either because they accidentally retrieve the wrong word or because they cannot retrieve the target word and deliberately produce a semantically related word as their compensatory strategy. In these cases, the substitution words are:
    - —semantically related to the targets.
    - —not necessarily phonologically easier for the child to produce than the targets.

Table 2-19. Early Grammatical Milestones

Stage	MLU	Age	Language Skills
pre-I	<1.0	<2;3	one-word utterances holophrases/formulas good prosody
I	1.1–2.0	1;6–2;3	"telegraphic"/contextual content words limited semantic relations
II	2–2.5	1;9–2;6	early bound morphemes irregular forms; prepositions early transformations
III	2.5–3	1;11–3;1	learn regulars and overgeneralize articles appear
IV	3.25–3.75	2;2–3;8	third-person forms
V	3.5–4.25	2;3–4;0	irregulars "relearned" auxiliaries, "be"

Source: Adapted from Owens (1996).

Table 2-20 can be used to document MLU and grammatical development. Morphemes and syntactic structures are listed in approximate order of acquisition on this form. At the top of the form, the child's MLU and age should be circled. If the circles do not line up, then the child's MLU is not age-appropriate. The range of utterance lengths within the language sample (e.g., from one to five morphemes per utterance) should be written in the "Range" section. On the bottom portion of the form, a check should be used to indicate any structures that the child uses consistently and correctly. If the structure is used inconsistently or inaccurately, an *e* should be placed on the line to indicate that this structure is emerging.

Table 2-20. Language Sample Form

Number of utterances:
Mean Length of Utterance (MLU):
Range of utterance lengths:
Circle the child's MLU and age in the chart below.

Stage	MLU	Age (in months)
Prelinguistic	0–1	8–12
Stage I	1.01–1.99	12–25
Stage II	2.00–2.59	26–30
Stage III	2.60–2.99	31–34
Stage IV	3.00–3.99	35–40
Stage V	4.00–4.50	41–46

This MLU is / is not appropriate for the child's chronological age. (Circle one.)

Morphology	**Syntax**
__ -ing	__ noun + verb + noun sentences
__ in, on	__ yes/no questions—intonation only
__ plural regular	__ simple negatives ("No want cookie")
__ plural irregular	__ yes/no questions—inverted auxiliary/copula
__ past irregular	__ negated auxiliary/copula (isn't, can't, etc.)
__ possessive "s"	__ adjectives
__ copula "be" (e.g., "She is pretty")	__ articles
__ articles	__ wh-questions—uninverted
__ past regular	__ pronouns
__ third-person singular regular	__ wh-questions—inverted auxiliary/copula
__ auxiliary verbs (e.g., "She is sleeping"; circle all that occur): be, have, can, do, will, might, should, could, would	__ compound sentences (and, because, etc.)
	__ comparative adjectives (-er, -est)
	__ adverbs (time, location, etc.)
	__ other:
__ other:	

KEY: √ = consistently used correctly
    e = emerging (inconsistently present or inconsistently correct) space left blank indicates
        child does not use this grammatical structure

Source: Bloom & Lahey (1978).

LITERACY

- WHO? Kindergarten and older children being assessed for literacy, with a prior diagnosis of phonological/phonetic delay/disorder or childhood apraxia.
- WHAT? Focus on literacy development.
- WHY? Certain aspects of literacy development may be difficult for children with childhood apraxia.
- LITERATURE RESOURCES: Frederickson, Frith, & Reason (1997); Robertson & Salter (1997); Stackhouse & Wells (1997, 2000); Stackhouse, Wells, Pascoe, & Rees (2002); Torgesen & Bryant (1994).

Areas for Assessment

Note: Areas that may be indicative of apraxia are in italics.

Sound-letter matching: Is the child able to answer the question, "What sound does this letter make?" for the letters of the alphabet?

Rhyming: Given a word, can the child provide a rhyming word (e.g., "pat-cat")?

*Onset-rhyme tasks (**alliteration**)—segmentation and blending:* Is the child able to build up or break down words into initial consonant versus the rest of the word?

Coda tasks—segmentation and blending: Is the child able to build up or break down words into the beginning of the word versus the final consonant?

Letter sequencing: Does the child write the letters in words in the proper sequence?

Word fluency (rapid automatic naming): Can the child orally name visually presented basic colors or shapes (or other very well-known items) rapidly, or are response times delayed?

Whole-part and part-whole reading and writing skills: Is the child able to build up or break down written words, sentences, and paragraphs?

Examples of some of these tasks, listed in approximate order of difficulty, are given below.

Tasks for Assessment

BASIC SEGMENTATION AND BLENDING TASKS
1. Choice: "What do you have in your yard—a birdhouse or a housebird?"
2. Fill in the blank: "A dog lives in a doghouse. A bird lives in a _____."
3. Compound segmentation: "If I take the 'house' off 'doghouse,' what's left?"
4. Compound blending: "If I put 'dog' in front of 'house,' what do I get?"

RHYMING TASKS

1. Multiple choice: "Which one rhymes with 'ball'—'fall' or 'bell'?"
2. List: "Tell me a word that rhymes with 'ball.'"

ONSET-RHYME TASKS (ALLITERATION)—SEGMENTATION AND BLENDING OF INITIAL CONSONANTS

1. Choice: "Which one starts with the same sound as 'cat'—'dog' or 'cup'?"
2. List: "Tell me a word that starts with the same sound as 'cat'."
3. Segmentation: "If I take the [k] sound off 'cat,' what's left?"
4. Blending: "If I say [k] and then [æt], what word does it make?"

CODA TASKS—SEGMENTATION AND BLENDING OF FINAL CONSONANTS

1. Multiple choice: "Which one ends with the same sound as 'moose'—'dog' or 'bus'?"
2. List: "Tell me a word that ends with the same sound as 'moose.'"
3. Segmentation: "If I take the [s] sound off 'moose,' what's left?"
4. Blending: "If I say 'moo' and then [s], what word does it make?"

PLAY CHARACTERISTICS

- WHO? Young children being assessed for phonological/phonetic and language delay/disorder with question of apraxia.
- WHAT? Focus on ability to carry out part-whole, whole-part, and **sequenced play routines.**
- WHY? Some children with apraxia have **ideomotor apraxia**: in children this manifests as difficulty with part-whole, whole-part, and/or sequenced play.
- LITERATURE RESOURCES: Linder (1993); Lowe & Costello (1976); Westby (1991).

Areas for Assessment

Note: Areas that may be indicative of apraxia are in italics.

Combinatorial play*: Ability to construct whole from parts (e.g., building with blocks) or to recognize parts of wholes (e.g., taking things apart).*

Pretend play: Ability to use one object to represent another (e.g., block as car). At a higher level, ability to use an imagined object to represent a real object (e.g., hand shaped as if holding a car, accompanied by engine noises).

*Sequenced or **embedded play routines**: Ability to pretend over larger domains (e.g., getting the baby ready for the babysitter: wake up, bathe, dress, feed, etc.); play routines have a plot or a theme.*

SECTION

3

TREATMENT

· ·

Unfortunately, clinical research into the treatment of childhood apraxia is sadly lacking. However, it is clear that there is no single recipe for treating this disorder, although there are some common principles that can be applied. Treatment must be tailored to the child's specific speech-language profile. Furthermore, children with apraxia tend not to follow a typical developmental course with respect to speech and language. Therefore, their strengths and weaknesses must be reassessed frequently, with intervention plans modified accordingly. An analytical, flexible approach to intervention planning is critical. The distinction between actions that require motor planning versus those that have become automatic through overlearning is central, as described by Ayres (1985):

> Planning requires thinking. If one has to think about actions, one is probably motor planning. If one does not have to think about them, the actions have probably become automatic and no longer require planning. . . . If therapy is designed to promote planning that requires thinking, then a variety of tasks that require thinking should be available. Once learned well, a task may no longer be therapeutic. (p. 24)

Speech-language pathologists and speech scientists have explored a variety of intervention theories and treatment approaches over the past several decades. We can benefit from their experience and insights as we investigate new perspectives and strategies.

Note: Children who are bilingual or bidialectal may require additional intervention modifications. See Goldstein (2000) for further information.

BASIC PRINCIPLES: TRADITIONAL APPROACHES

- WHO? Children with childhood apraxia of speech.
- WHAT? Basic principles that are common to many traditional intervention approaches.
- WHY? As stated by Love (1993), "the consistent commentary that apraxic children fare poorly in therapy and require extensive and extended intervention does not speak well for this [traditional] approach without qualification" (p. 200). However, these traditional approaches form the foundations of many current approaches. Knowledge of approaches that have been used in the past can help us to both avoid pitfalls inherent in those approaches and prevent us from reinventing wheels that have already carried us far.
- LITERATURE RESOURCES: Bashir, Grahamjones, & Bostwick (1984); Caruso & Strand (1999); Chumpelik (1984); Crary (1993); Hall, Jordan, & Robin (1993); Haynes (1985); Helfrich-Miller (1984); Lowe (1993); Rosenbeck, Hansen, Baughman, & Lemme (1974; cited by Crary 1993); Yoss & Darley (1974).

Traditional approaches to apraxia intervention include the following recommendations.

Emphasize movement sequences.

Use intensive, systematic drill with many repetitions.

Use a limited number of stimuli per goal and per session.

Facilitate production using visual, rhythmic, prosodic, and motor cues (multiple modalities).

Begin with imitation; sustained vowels and consonants are often suggested as a starting point.

Teach **carrier phrases**, for example, "I wanna _____" or "Let's _____."

Encourage self-monitoring.

Encourage slowed rate.

Use **touch cues** to increase articulatory awareness (see Supplementary Strategies).

Use a phonetic hierarchy of treatment targets, from consonants and vowels in isolation, through syllables and words, to phrases and sentences.

Note: Teaching sounds in isolation is not recommended by Velleman and K. Strand; E. Strand and Skinder; Square; or Marquardt and Sussman. Although there are anecdotal reports that it is easier for children with apraxia to learn sounds in isolation, this does not appear to carry over to the use of the same sounds in syllables and words. Thus, it is not the best use of therapy time.

Teach compensatory strategies, such as equal stress, pauses, and **intrusive schwa**s in consonant clusters

   Note: This is not recommended by Velleman and Shriberg (1999) and others, as it tends to yield very unnatural prosody that may then persist and have to be untrained at a later time.

Select some easily attainable objectives to ensure that the child experiences success.

Increase oral sensory awareness using tactile stimulation (massage, brushing, tastes, etc.) to the oral area.

Introduce a core vocabulary of functional words to increase communicative efficacy.

BASIC PRINCIPLES: DYNAMIC MOTOR APPROACHES

- WHO? Children with childhood apraxia of speech.
- WHAT? Basic principles that apply to all treatment goals, at all levels.
- WHY? In a newer variation of the motor approach, E. Strand and Skinder (1999) suggest "integral stimulation treatment." Marquardt and Sussman (1991) propose taking advantage of facilitating phonetic contexts. Square (1999) recommends that treatment focus on establishing sensorimotor schemas for recognizing, recalling, and responding to speech production routines. All three discourage training of isolated consonant or vowel sounds and encourage production of syllable and word shapes.
- LITERATURE RESOURCES: Chumpelik (1984); Davis & Velleman (2000); Hayden & Square (1994); Marquardt & Sussman (1991); Square (1999); E. Strand & Skinder (1999).

E. Strand and Skinder: Integral stimulation:
- Help the child understand that the goal of the session is to practice movements.
- Provide opportunities for early success to maximize trust and motivation.
- Use varied body positions, prosodic contours, and props to maintain attention.
- Emphasize **mass practice** (many repetitions of a few targets) for more severe cases; **distributed practice** (repetitions of more targets with a common gestural basis) for moderate cases.
- Begin with direct imitation of the word at a slowed rate.
- If the child is successful, continue direct imitation until the child can imitate accurately at a normal speech rate, with varying prosody. Then, add a gradually increasing delay after the model.
- If the child is not successful at slowed-rate imitation, provide simultaneous productions: child and therapist produce the word together at a slowed rate. Once the child can do simultaneous productions at a normal rate with varying prosody, go back to direct imitation.
- If the child is not successful with simultaneous productions alone, add tactile cues and slow rate even further.

Marquardt and Sussman:
- Stabilize vowels and consonants already in the child's repertoire.
- Select additional targets from early developing sounds whose articulation is visible.
- Select sounds that contrast with each other to maximize communicative efficacy.
- Use phonetic context to facilitate production.
- **Multimodal** (visual, tactile) **inputs** are emphasized.
- Movement sequences and maintaining syllabic integrity are emphasized.

Square: Prompts for Restructuring Oral Muscular Phonetic Targets
- Clinician's hands provide support and tactile cues to the oral musculature.
- Establish postural support for trunk, neck, and head control.
- Suppress abnormal **oral-motor reflex**es.
- Establish **phonatory control** (ability to voice) for two to three seconds.
- Establish control of vertical jaw movements, while inhibiting horizontal and anterior-posterior movements.
- Establish control over **grading of** jaw **movements**: different degrees of opening for different vowels.
- Establish symmetrical, coordinated movements of the upper and lower lips for lip rounding and retraction.
- Establish control of coordinated movements of the tongue, including anterior-posterior movements, raising-lowering movements, and contraction.
- Retain control of the above for longer streams of speech.
- Retain control of the above while normalizing rate and intonation.

BASIC PRINCIPLES: "LINGUISTIC" APPROACHES

- WHO? Children with childhood apraxia of speech.
- WHAT? Basic principles that apply to all treatment goals, at all levels.
- WHY? In the view of Velleman and K. Strand (1994, 1998), childhood apraxia is a disorder of hierarchical organization that especially affects sequencing and dynamic planning. According to Crary (1984), symptoms may range from those that reflect "executive" deficits (difficulty in carrying out motor plans, exemplified by struggle and distortions) to those that reflect planning deficits (difficulty in devising motor plans, exemplified by sequencing errors and language errors). They advocate that treatments for all aspects of the disorder should reflect these ideas. However, these principles, like those above, are based upon theory and clinical experience. They have not been verified through careful empirical research.
- LITERATURE RESOURCES: Marquardt & Sussman (1991); Crary (1993); Velleman & K. Strand (1994, 1998).

The following principles are emphasized in linguistic approaches, especially Velleman and Strand (1994, 1998).

Both automaticity (a functional core vocabulary) and flexibility (the ability to plan and carry out novel speech sequences) should be addressed. Therefore, drill alone is insufficient as it addresses only automaticity.

Old forms (syllable or word shapes) with new content (sounds); new forms with old content.

The hardest task for children with CAS is not the sounds themselves, but putting them together into a smooth, fluent utterance. Therefore:
- The main focus of treatment should be syllable structure control and organization.
- Treatment must occur within a variety of dynamic linguistic contexts. That is, the clinician should be sure to vary the social and/or linguistic contexts enough that they don't become entirely predictable and, therefore, automatic. Practice under slightly dissimilar circumstances is more challenging because it requires ongoing motor planning and thus, it is more likely to enhance generalization. However, note that change should be carefully controlled: only one dimension of the context (e.g., social or linguistic) should be varied at a time.

Working on sounds in isolation is often easier for children with apraxia, but does not carry over to syllables and words. A sound-by-sound treatment plan that emphasizes phoneme production in isolation prior to moving to words and phrases does *not* address the hierarchical dynamic movement problem in CAS. It is more efficient to begin at the syllable level. If the child has difficulty producing full syllables (a consonant combined with a vowel), simple words or syllables composed of a vowel and a glottal consonant (e.g., "uh-oh", "ha ha", "hey", "hi", etc.) or of a vowel and a glide (e.g., "wow", "yay", "whee", "whoa") are often accessible, especially those that have emotional content (as do those in the examples given here). If isolated phonemes are to be addressed, those that carry meaning as such (e.g., [u:] or [o:] to express surprise or awe, [m:] to mean "yummy," or [ʃ] to mean "be quiet") should be targeted, as they will increase communicative efficacy.

Auditory discrimination training does *not* address the core problem, although some subtle auditory discrimination difficulties may become apparent and require intervention in mid-childhood.

There are two critical aspects of motor sequencing, both of which should be integrated into therapy activities whenever possible:
- Determining the order of the elements ("Which sound do I say first?")
- Figuring out how to get from one to the other ("How do I get to the next articulatory position from this one?")

Since CAS is a dynamic disorder, system fatigue is a problem. Therefore:
- Frequent, short sessions with breaks are most successful.
- Focus on only one new aspect of speech production at a time, as simultaneous multiple changes (e.g., a new sound in a new position in a new social context) can be overwhelming.
- Work with occupational therapy on **sensory integration** issues, and with occupational and physical therapists on non-oral/non-speech motor planning issues.

SUPPLEMENTAL STRATEGIES

- WHO? Children with childhood apraxia of speech.
- WHAT? Supplemental approaches providing tactile, rhythmic, or gestural cues to the client.
- WHY? Children with childhood apraxia of speech may lack the **sensorimotor feedback loops** or sensorimotor rhythmic foundation necessary to plan, monitor, and self-correct during speech production. Supplementary strategies include tactile, rhythmic, or gestural cues to enhance these skills.
- LITERATURE RESOURCES: Bashir, Grahamjones, & Bostwick (1984); Chumpelik (1984); Davis & Velleman (2000); Hall, Jordan, & Robin (1993); Hayden & Square (1994); Helfrich-Miller (1984); Square (1994, 1999).

Tactile Cues
- Touch cues: Bashir, Grahamjones, and Bostwick
  —Tactile cues for place of articulation of eight English speech sounds.
  — Intended to be used dynamically, to signal speech movement sequences.
  —However, no cues suggested for vowels.
  —Teach phonemes in the following order: /b/, /d/, /g/, /s/, /f/, /n/, /ʃ/, /l/.
  —Training proceeds in three stages:
    (1) Nonsense syllable drills
    (2) Monosyllabic and polysyllabic words, emphasizing contrasts in place, manner, and voicing
    (3) Controlled multiword utterances, then spontaneous speech
- Prompts for Restructuring Oral Muscular Phonetic Targets: Hayden and Square
  —Built upon Moto-Kinesthetic Speech Training (Young & Stichfield-Hawk, 1955).
  —Manual stimulation of the muscles of the face using varying degrees of pressure and timing to give the child the feeling of the desired movement sequence.
  —Head, jaw, thoracic region may also be manually stimulated or supported.
  —Hierarchical program of movement training: See "Newer Motor Approaches," above.
  —Focus on dynamic movement sequences for production of functional words and phrases.

Rhythmic/Melodic Methods
- Rhythmic repetition and alternation of single syllables: Velleman and K. Strand (1994, 1998); see "Practicing the Scales" in "Suggested Treatment Protocol" and also "Training Motor Planning Flexibility."
- **Melodic Intonation Therapy** (adapted for children by Helfrich-Miller, 1984): speech production facilitated by rhythms or tunes.
  —gradual increase in output length.
  —gradual increase in phonemic complexity.
  —gradual decrease in reliance on clinician's cues.
  —gradual decrease in reliance on intonation patterns.
  —Helfrich-Miller recommends use of signed English as a pacing cue and to highlight grammatical structure.
  —Others (e.g., Smith & Engel, 1984) recommend tapping, as is used with adults.

Gestural Cues
- Designed to provide supplemental visual/tactile information about articulatory movements and postures.
- Incorporated as one component of other approaches, for example, touch cues, Melodic Intonation Therapy.
- Adapted Cueing Therapy (Klick, 1984, 1994):
  —Continuous hand motion at the clinician's face level.
  —Represent movement patterns of the articulators and air flow through the vocal tract.
- Cued Speech (Cornett, 1972):
  —Initially developed to supplement lip reading for people who are deaf.
  —Eight hand shapes.
  —Four hand positions at various positions on and around the face.
  —Signal articulatory features, including voicing and nasality.
- Jordan's Gestures (Jordan 1988, 1991):
  —One or both hands required, depending on phone.
  —Represent contact points of phone.
  —Represent manner of production of phone, including voicing.
  —Represent required articulatory movements.

SUGGESTED TREATMENT PROTOCOL: OVERVIEW

- WHO? Children with apraxia.
- WHAT? Format for the typical hierarchically oriented speech-language therapy session.
- WHY? Sessions should be divided into short segments. Each part addresses a different aspect of the child's communication disorder. Each segment will be described in more detail later in this section.
- LITERATURE RESOURCES: Velleman & K. Strand (1994, 1998).

Velleman and Strand (1994, 1998) recommend the following treatment protocol.

Warm-up: Stimulation and movement to increase awareness and flexibility.
- Increase oral-motor/body awareness and muscle tone via **tactile stimulation**. (Consult occupational therapist if unsure of appropriate activities for particular children.)
- Warm up the muscles and the motor-planning system via imitation of body and/or oral-motor sequences. May be done within play or music contexts.
- Tune up: Practice producing varied pitch patterns, loudness levels, and rhythms. Use either well-established speech patterns or non-speech vocalizations or body movements. (May be combined with the above.)

Practicing the scales: Syllable/word/phrase sequence drill activities for flexibility. Establish consistent connected syllable productions from within the child's repertoire. With young/severely affected children, it is preferable to use meaningful words in order to expand their communicative repertoires while addressing the motor-planning problem. For older children, nonsense syllables/words may be appropriate, especially if they have difficulty breaking well-established incorrect patterns of production of familiar words.
Note: These activities should be based upon phonetic elements already under the child's articulatory control.

- Ability to produce repeated syllable sequences (e.g., babababa).
- Ability to anticipate articulatory change in syllable sequences (e.g., babababa, badabada).

Learning the song: Meaningful single-word/phrase activities to provide automaticity for a core group of words/phrases and increase communicative effectiveness.
- Functional phrases, rhymes, and songs learned to the level of automaticity.
- Ability to plug in variations within a well-known frame (e.g., "Let's ___"; "On his farm he had a ___").

Changing the song: Combining automatic elements flexibly into a variety of smooth, fluent utterances. Use:

- Picture cues.
- Rhythmic cues.
- Change one word at a time in a known sentence frame—not necessarily from the same "slot." (E.g., "I'll see you tomorrow," "I'll see you later," "I'll call you later," "I'll call him later," etc.)
- Increase length and complexity of sentences.
- Provide explicit practice of various intonation and stress patterns. For younger children, model without calling attention to the nature of the pattern. For older children with some **metalinguistic awareness**, increase awareness as well as production of suprasegmentals.

SOCIAL CONSIDERATIONS

- WHO? Children with high frustration levels, resulting behavior management problems, excessive shyness/withdrawal, and/or family member cited as interpreter.
- WHAT? Goals directed toward immediate improvement in communicative effectiveness.
- WHY? Due to their speech-language deficits, children with this social profile are not able to experience normal communicative interactions and are thereby missing important opportunities for learning critical social skills.
- LITERATURE RESOURCES: Kaufman (1998, 2001); Velleman & K. Strand (1994, 1998).

In cases in which children present with high frustration levels, resulting behavior management problems, excessive shyness/withdrawal, and/or a family member cited as interpreter, a two-pronged approach is required to increase communicative efficacy:

Identification of core social concepts that this particular child needs to be able to express, such as:
- An appropriate, conventional way to say "No!"
- "More"; this concept can be used flexibly in a wide variety of situations.
- Names of siblings, pets, and other significant others (including the child herself!).
- A very frustrated child may benefit from being taught to express her frustration by approximating (or signing) "Mad!"
- A child with several siblings who tease him might benefit from being taught to approximate, "Dummy!" back at them (J. Johnston, personal communication, 1990).
- A child with a grabby sibling or classmate would greatly appreciate being taught to approximate, "Mine!" or "Gimme."
- Many of these expressions are not among parents' or teachers' top-ten lists, but they have a real impact on the child's frustration level, and may significantly reduce tantrums or withdrawal behaviors. Furthermore, they are words that are commonly used by young children who are developing normally. Thus, they will contribute to normalizing the child's social development.

Selection of word targets for expressing these core concepts based upon the child's current phonetic and phonotactic capabilities:
- Sounds that the child is able to produce.
- Word shapes that the child is able to produce.
- Word positions in which the child currently produces those sounds.
- See "Training Automaticity."

These are not phonological goals. They are social goals, intended to maximize the child's ability to interact communicatively with peers as well as adults. Rapid success is critical to the child's social development. Therefore, word targets should be as easy as possible for the child to produce.

Kaufman (1998, 2001) provides a therapy kit that facilitates selection of word approximations for children who cannot produce a particular word accurately. For example, she suggests that the child might produce "animal" as "ana-mo" or "amo"; "time" as "t-ime" or "tah-eem" or "tah-m"; "toot" as "t-oot" or "too-t."

Note: One drawback to Kaufman's **synthesis** recommendations ("t-oot," "tah-eem," etc.) is that they do not preserve the integrity of the words or syllables that the child is attempting. Children with apraxia have difficulty integrating sounds into a word; the focus should be on training the child to produce such transitions.

COMMUNICATIVE MEANS

> - WHO? Any child with communicative delays.
> - WHAT? Priorities to improve communication.
> - WHY? Intervention must start at the child's current level of functioning. Children with apraxia may make progress in very small steps. Therefore, careful planning requires an in-depth awareness of the child's current communicative means and strategies.
> - LITERATURE RESOURCES: Davis & Velleman (2000); Frost & Bondy (1994); Velleman & K. Strand (1994, 1998).

Depending on the child's communicative level, various strategies can be used to increase her or his communicative means.

Few, immature, and/or unintelligible vocalizations
- Teach child to use alternative communication strategies to reduce frustration:
    —gestures
    —leading
    —mime
    —sign
    —pictures (such as the Picture Exchange Communication System, an augmentative communication system in which the child hands a picture to the listener as his or her turn in the conversation or in order to request the object or action pictured)
- Model words and meaningful vocalizations that are easier for children with apraxia to approximate:
    —words with distinctive pitch patterns (e.g., uh-oh, wow, whee, yay).
    —words with strong emotional meaning (e.g., uh-oh, wow, whee, yay).
    —words that can be paired with actions (e.g., whee, hi, oops).
    —words with very early consonants (e.g., [h], glides) and simple syllable shapes (e.g., hi, uh-oh, wow, whee, yay).
    —sound effects: animal noises, vehicle noises, etc.
- Accept such words and sound effects as meaningful (e.g., "meow" is initially accepted to mean "cat").
- See "Training Automaticity."

Many unintelligible words:

- Decrease use of idiosyncratic, non-conventional words (or signs, or gestures) *at a manageable rate.* A child with many non-conventional words, signs, or gestures typically relies upon these means of communication. Therefore, the majority of those that are understood by family members or others familiar with the child should continue to serve that function at the same time as a few selected words are targeted for more conventional production, via encouragement of consistency and discouragement of homonymy (described below).
- Encourage consistent production of words within the child's expressive vocabulary. For example, if the child uses "dada," "papa," and "tata" all to mean "daddy," ask the family/other significant people in the child's life to choose only one form that will be accepted with that meaning. Other forms will be treated as nonsense words.
- Discourage homonymy. For example, if the child uses "tata" to mean "daddy," "potato," and "bye-bye," ask the family/other significant people in the child's life to choose one meaning that will be accepted for that form. Other apparent meanings will be treated as if misunderstood ("Why are you calling daddy a potato?").

No word combinations

- Encourage combinations of oral word plus sign, oral word plus gesture, or oral word plus pictures, where the sign/gesture/picture adds meaning rather than reinforcing the oral word.
- Encourage other combinatorial activities, especially sequences of pretend play.

NON-SPEECH ORAL-MOTOR OR ORAL-SENSORY SYMPTOMS

- WHO? Children whose symptoms affect non-speech oral activities as well as speech activities.
- WHAT? Techniques to address **non-speech** oral-motor and oral-sensory symptoms.
- WHY? *Non-speech therapy activities will not improve a child's speech. Activities that address speech directly are critical for that purpose.* However, some children with apraxia have non-speech oral deficits as well. The speech-language pathologist can be one member of the team remediating oral-sensory or oral-motor feeding difficulties that interfere with non-speech activities (feeding, toothbrushing, etc.). Furthermore, non-speech oral-motor and/or oral-sensory therapy may provide a good warm-up for speech therapy in some cases, because it may increase the child's oral awareness and tone the oral musculature in the process.
- LITERATURE RESOURCES: Bahr (2001); Boshart (1998); Forrest (2002); Mackie (1996a, b); Morris (1997a, b, c); Ripley, Daines, & Barrett (1997).

Note: Traditionally in the literature the term "non-verbal" is used rather than the term "non-speech." This usage implies that one who does not speak is not verbal. However, the production of sign language, written language, and computer-generated language are all *verbal* non-speech activities. Therefore, the more precise term, "non-speech" is used here.

Strategies for addressing non-speech oral-motor or oral-sensory symptoms include the following.

Consult with an occupational therapist.

Use tactile stimulation to increase oral awareness (if the child is hyposensitive) or to increase tolerance (if the child is hypersensitive).
- In some cases, tactile stimulation to the body may need to be introduced before the child will be able to accept stimulation to the face and mouth.
- Work from cheeks to jaw to lips.
- Use only firm, slow pressure for a child who is hypersensitive.
- Use massage and light, quick strokes as well as firm touch for a child who is hyposensitive.
- Inside the mouth, work from teeth/gums to inside cheeks, tongue (tip, blade, then sides), hard palate.
- Tell the child what you are going to do before and as you do it.
- Provide objects with a variety of textures for oral stimulation (Nuk, Infa-Dent, Hand & Foot Teethers, Gummy Yummy, Humbug massager, plastic tubing to chew on).
- Encourage the child's own exploration of his or her mouth with *clean* hands to increase the child's awareness of the articulators.

Oral-motor treatment
- Imitation or production of specific postures is often facilitated by:
  - —Use of a mirror.
  - —Accompanying gestures (e.g., opening hand to accompany opening mouth)—if limb apraxia is not a factor.
  - —Visual and tactile cues, including food-based devices such as lollipops and play-based devices such as puppets or children's lipstick.
  - —For older children, verbal cues describing the desired movement (e.g., "Put your tongue higher") or pictures of the mouth in the correct position.
- Imitation or production of sequences should be the main focus. Postures that the child can already produce form the basis for such sequences. Again, visual, tactile, and verbal cues are often helpful.

Feeding
- Consult with an occupational therapist and other feeding team members.
- Use tactile stimulation to increase oral awareness (if the child is hyposensitive) or to increase tolerance (if the child is hypersensitive) immediately before introducing food; see above for examples.
- Gradually increase the child's repertoire of foods, introducing only one change at a time: texture, combination of textures, taste, and temperature.
- Introduce changes "recreationally" first, before family incorporates them into meals.
- Encourage food play; many children like to determine the texture and temperature of the food first with their hands before putting it in their mouths.

OTHER SENSORIMOTOR DEFICITS

- WHO? Children with other sensorimotor deficits, such as limb or body apraxia.
- WHAT? Questions and suggestions for working together with other members of the team to minimize negative effects of sensorimotor deficits on progress in speech-language therapy and maximize the child's overall progress.
- WHY? People focus better when their bodies are comfortable; they speak better when their posture facilitates breath support and normalizes muscle tone. Sensorimotor deficits have the potential to interfere indirectly with successful speech-language development.
- LITERATURE RESOURCE: Ayres (1985).

Motor planning difficulties, especially for action sequences (hands, whole body)
- Ideally, work with an occupational therapist or physical therapist, or
- Schedule speech-language therapy sessions immediately following occupational therapy or physical therapy, or
- Observe the occupational or physical therapist during sessions to learn appropriately stimulating action sequences, or
- Ask an occupational therapist or physical therapist for an appropriate hierarchy of actions that could be paired with verbal cues during the warm-up portion of the session.

Mild to moderate sensory hypersensitivity, hyposensitivity, or both in different areas of the face and/or body
- Ideally, work with an occupational therapist, or
- Schedule speech-language therapy sessions immediately following occupational therapy, or
- Ask an occupational therapist for an appropriate hierarchy of sensory stimulation/ awareness or **desensitization** activities that could be paired with verbal cues during the warm-up portion of the session.

Mildly low muscle tone (*Note:* Extreme tone differences usually accompany a more purely motor-based disorder than apraxia, such as cerebral palsy.)
- Ideally, work with an occupational therapist or physical therapist, or
- Schedule speech-language therapy sessions immediately following occupational therapy or physical therapy, or
- Ask an occupational therapist or physical therapist for an appropriate hierarchy of activities for improving muscle tone that could be paired with verbal cues during the warm-up portion of the session.

SPEECH ORAL-MOTOR AND ORAL-SENSORY FACTORS

- WHO? Children whose speech is directly affected by oral-motor and/or oral-sensory factors.
- WHAT? Strategies for improving speech motor skills and sensory awareness for speech.
- WHY? Motor planning for speech, including awareness of the positions of the articulators, is a common deficit in children with apraxia of speech.
- LITERATURE RESOURCES: Bahr (2001); Forrest (2002); E. Strand & Skinder (1999).

Strategies for improving speech motor skills and sensory awareness for speech including the following.

Hyposensitivity, hypersensitivity, poor muscle tone: See "Non-Speech Oral-Motor or Oral-Sensory Symptoms" and "Other Sensorimotor Deficits" in the earlier sections above.

Difficulty organizing and sequencing segments in a variety of dynamic patterns
- Establish consistent connected syllable productions from within the child's repertoire, ranging from repetitions of the same syllable to sequences that vary articulatory positions (e.g., from front to back—[bʌdʌgʌ] or "buttercup"—or vice versa—[gʌdʌbʌ] or "go to bed").
- With young/severely affected children, use meaningful words; for older children, nonsense syllables/words may be appropriate.
- See "Training Motor Planning Flexibility."

TRAINING AUTOMATICITY

- WHO? Children with little automatic social language.
- WHAT? A suggested sequence of goals for teaching a core set of automatic words or utterances.
- WHY? A child cannot wait for improved motor-planning flexibility before being able to communicate basic ideas and feelings. Many people with apraxia find that the more urgent their communicative need, the harder it is for them to produce the desired words. Words that have been practiced repeatedly in low-stress situations, however, can become automatic: planning is no longer required in order to produce them. Thus, a core vocabulary of overlearned words and phrases will allow the child to enter the world of successful communication.
- LITERATURE RESOURCES: Davis & Velleman (2000); Velleman & K. Strand (1994, 1998).

Velleman and Strand (1994, 1998) offer the following guidelines for increasing a child's repertoire of automatic speech utterances.

Choose words and utterances with strong social value to the particular child in certain situations. These may not be the same words that the parents or teachers want the child to be able to produce (e.g., "bathroom" may be at the top of the adults' list, but not the child's). See "Social Considerations."

Don't bother working on words that express ideas the child can already successfully communicate in other (non-speech) modalities, such as "yes" and "no" for a child who can nod or shake her head with ease.

Encourage the child to use sound effects to express meanings when this can be done with success (e.g., "meow" is accepted to mean "cat"; therefore, "cat" is not an appropriate objective for immediate automaticity training for a child who can consistently say "meow"). Instead, target words or concepts that the child has no way of expressing.

Model words and utterances that are easier for children with apraxia to approximate, including words with distinctive pitch patterns, words with very early developing consonants, words with strong emotional meaning, and words that can be paired with actions. (See "Communicative Means.")

Enlist as many school staff, family members, and other significant others as possible to model the same words and utterances, and to accept the child's closest approximations.

Teach new words in facilitating social, linguistic, and motor contexts:
- In verbal routines: songs, rhymes, social routines (e.g., "good morning"), academic routines (e.g., counting, reciting months), prayers, and so on.
- In unison situations, where there is very little communicative pressure because everyone is saying or singing the same thing.
- With a puppet or other toy "doing the talking" to reduce direct communicative pressure on the child.
- In fill-in-the-blank contexts, such as the ends of lines in repetitive songs, predictable books, and the like (e.g., "The wheels on the bus go ____"; "E - I - E - I - ___"; "Duck, duck, ____"; "I'll huff and I'll ___"; etc.). Gradually expand from contexts in which there is only one fill-in option (such as those listed above) to contexts in which there is a choice (e.g., "and on his farm he had a ____").
- In utterance frames that normally developing children really use (e.g., "Let's ___"; "More ____, please"; "MY ___"; "Stop ____"; and even "Gimme ____").
- With accompanying motor movements ("Head, Tummy, Knees and Toes"), if the child does not have co-occurring body apraxia.

Note: The "Time to Sing" CD, recorded by members of the Pittsburgh Symphony Orchestra for the Center for Creative Play (http://www.center4creativeplay.org), includes many popular children's songs arranged by composer Michael Moricz (former Music Director of "Mister Rogers' Neighborhood," and current Resident Composer and Company Pianist of the Pittsburgh Ballet Theatre) at a slower pace to make it easier for children with apraxia or other speech problems to sing along.

Take advantage of every opportunity to model these words and phrases, or to give the child a chance to practice them in non-stressful/risk-free contexts.

Caution parents not to put the child on show to produce new words for Grandma, for example, until the child has achieved automatic control over these productions.

Do not make correct production of these words a price for obtaining something the child wants or needs (e.g., "You can't have it unless you say it"). Automaticity training should be fun and rewarding.

TRAINING MOTOR-PLANNING FLEXIBILITY

- WHO? Children with difficulty organizing and sequencing segments in a variety of dynamic patterns.
- WHAT? A suggested sequence of goals.
- WHY? In order to train speech motor planning, the speech-language pathologist must start with the child's current status and work up systematically to more difficult sequences.
- LITERATURE RESOURCES: Bashir et al. (1984); Davis & Velleman (2000); Kirkpatrick et al. (1990); Velleman & K. Strand (1994, 1998).

Speech motor-planning flexibility should be trained in the following sequence.

Ability to produce repeated phonetic sequences, beginning with "easy" consonants and vowels:
- CV forms with consistency of consonant and vowel production across four to 10 repetitions (baa-baa-baa-baa, etc.). Vary consonant or vowel types (place or manner of articulation) as the child's phonetic repertoire permits, changing only one segment at a time (consonant *or* vowel). Maintain the same CV across all repetitions in each instance.
  Examples: ba-ba-ba-ba-ba, then da-da-da-da-da, or
  ba-ba-ba-ba-ba, then bee-bee-bee-bee-bee
- Repetition of more difficult phonotactic shapes (CVC and beyond), in the same manner. This objective should be addressed in conjunction with those below. See "A Hierarchy of Phonotactic (Syllable and Word Shape) Difficulty" (p.76) for guidance in choosing an appropriate sequence of phonotactic shapes.

Ability to anticipate articulatory change in repeated phonetic sequences:
- Minimally change CV productions in response to visual (picture or letters) cue after four to nine repetitions (e.g., baa-baa-baa-baa-boo-boo-boo-boo). Change either the vowel or the consonant, not both, at this stage. Target vowels and consonants should be sounds that are already in the child's phonetic repertoire. Also, they must be sounds that the child produces distinctly enough that changes can be detected. (For example, if both /ɑ/ and /o/ are pronounced as [ʌ], no vowel change is actually occurring.) Usually, stops and **corner vowels** ([i, ɑ, u]) are good places to begin.
- Minimally change CV production (consonant or vowel) in an alternating sequence of four to 10 repetitions (e.g., baa-boo-baa-boo, etc.).
- Minimally change CV production (consonant or vowel) in randomly alternating sequences of four to 10 repetitions (e.g., baa-baa-boo-baa-boo-boo, etc.).
- Continue with a variety of consonant and vowel types (place and manner of articulation, e.g., labial stops, labial nasal, labiovelar glide, low back vowel, low front vowel, etc.), always using pairs within the child's phonetic repertoire that differ by only one consonant or one vowel.
- Continue with increasingly more significant changes required (e.g., both consonant and vowel changed), and/or with increasing numbers of different CV words.
- Continue with more challenging phonotactic shapes (CVC and beyond). See "A Hierarchy of Phonotactic (Syllable and Word Shape) Difficulty" (p.76) for guidance on choosing an appropriate sequence of phonotactic shapes.

Possible strategies and activities:

- Play routines: perform actions with multiples of the same toy or type of toy, such as setting the table, sorting laundry, lining up animals to enter a toy barn, and so on, labeling the items as you perform the action ("bowl bowl bowl," "sock sock sock," "moo moo moo moo," etc.). Once the listing/labeling routine is established, pause immediately before performing the last action and producing the last repetition; wait for the child to say the target word, then do the action. This provides the child the opportunity to fill in the blank. Initially, it may be necessary to mouthe the word or quietly pronounce the first sound along with the child to facilitate the production. Gradually, shift more and more responsibility for producing the entire sequence onto the child. *Note:* If the target word has a final consonant, its production should not be required initially. Similarly, more difficult phonemes (such as [s]) may or may not be produced accurately. The goal is for the child to produce a sequence of CV syllables smoothly and *consistently*; if the child produces "sock" as [dɑ], that same pronunciation should be repeated by the child as each sock is handled. The clinician, of course, always models the correct form of the word, but not judgmentally.
- Book reading (e.g., counting books): repeat the name of the object ("ball, ball, ball") instead of counting the number of objects in a manner similar to that described for play routines.
- The **ba-ba board**: Paste the same set of pictures (e.g., Mayer-Johnson pictures) representing the target syllables into several 3 x 5 inch spiral notebooks. Then, line the notebooks up on the table (or, hang them over a hanging file drawer frame), flipping pages as appropriate. Group pictures phonetically. For example, the first section of each stops book includes syllables with initial [b]: "bee, baa, boo, bow, boy, buy, bay." Thus, the entire row of stops books can be lined up and turned to the "bee" page, for example, for the child to point to and name one by one. The next section in the stops book could be [d] syllables, in the same sequence of vowels (as possible, given that some syllables will not be picturable): "dee," (no picture for [dɑ]), "dew, doe/dough, day." The voiceless stops sections (usually at the end of the stops book, as initial voiceless stops are more difficult than initial voiced stops) would include [p] with: "pea, pa, Pooh, pie, pay, paw, pow"; and so on. Other sets of books would include glide-initial syllables, fricative-initial syllables, and so on. For older children who have some literacy skills, syllables can be written out instead. Be careful to spell the syllables/words not in International Phonetic Alphabet (IPA) but as they would be spelled in English orthography!
- Tactile cues used dynamically: Model the transition of articulatory postures via the transition of hand postures (see "Supplemental Strategies").
- Rhyming games—at the CVC level: bat, hat, cat, pat . . .
- For more advanced children: *Moving Across Syllables* program (Kirkpatrick et al., 1990): a systematic program targeting movement patterns by place of articulation (e.g., bilabial to velar, as in "bag"; velar to bilabial, as in "gab").

A HIERARCHY OF PHONOTACTIC (SYLLABLE AND WORD SHAPE) DIFFICULTY

- WHO? Children with difficulty organizing and sequencing segments in a variety of dynamic patterns.
- WHAT? A suggested sequence of goals based upon phonotactic (syllable and word shape) difficulty.
- WHY? In order to train speech motor planning, the speech-language pathologist must start with the child's current status and work up systematically to more difficult sequences.
- LITERATURE RESOURCE: Davis & Velleman (2000); Velleman (1998, 2002).

Children with apraxia often appear to dance to a different drummer; they do not necessarily follow more typical developmental progressions. Therefore, it is especially important with these clients that the speech-language pathologist probe for stimulability before embarking upon the next goal. The child may be ready for a goal that is typically more difficult than the one that is anticipated to be next in the sequence. For example, a child with apraxia may master initial consonant clusters before final consonants or before two-syllable words. The following sequence, therefore, is a rough guideline.

Simple open syllables (CV)
- If the child has no "true" consonants, begin with glides and glottals—"whee!", "hi", "yay", "Wow!", and the like.

Reduplicated open syllables (CVCV—same syllable repeated, as in "bye-bye").

Harmonized non-reduplicated disyllabic forms: CVCV with either
- Matching vowels but different consonants, as in "TV", or
- Matching consonants but different vowels, as in "baby."

Non-harmonized, non-reduplicated disyllabic forms: CVCV with different consonants and different vowels, as in "buddy."

Harmonized closed syllables (CVC—same consonant repeated, as in "bib").

Non-harmonized closed syllables (CVC—different consonant, as in "dog").

CVCVC words:
- Same consonants and vowels
- Different consonants
- Different vowels
- Different consonants and vowels

Words with initial, medial, and/or final clusters.

PATTERN-BASED APPROACHES
TO PHONOLOGICAL INTERVENTION

> • WHO? Children with apraxia whose speech errors fall into patterns, such as final consonant deletion, fronting, affrication, voicing, and so on.
> • WHAT? Suggested guidelines for using a pattern-based approach (such as phonological process therapy) with children with apraxia.
> • WHY? Like other children with phonological disorders, children with apraxia often demonstrate error patterns. That is, their errors typically do not affect one consonant or vowel in an apparently random manner that is unrelated to other errors in their speech.
> • LITERATURE RESOURCES: Hodson & Paden (1991); Stoel-Gammon, Stone-Goldman, & Glaspey (2002).

Although the vast majority of speech-language pathologists are well acquainted with pattern-based approaches to phonological therapy (such as process therapy), the basic assumptions and strategies for these approaches are given below, along with a few suggestions for applying these approaches to children with apraxia of speech.

Basic assumptions underlying pattern-based approaches to phonological therapy:
- Children's errors fall into several common patterns, commonly referred to as
  —**processes** if the focus is on the difference between the adult form of the word and the child's error form (e.g., saying [dɪt] for "fish" is referred to as **stopping** because the target fricatives are produced as stops).
  —**constraints** if the focus is on the phonetic feature or phonotactic structure that the child appears to be avoiding (e.g., saying [dɪt] for "fish" is referred to as "*fricative" because the child appears to be avoiding the production of fricatives as such).
- It is more effective and efficient to target an entire error pattern at once (e.g., stopping of all fricatives) than to target each instance of that error pattern one at a time (e.g., teaching each fricative, one by one).
- Over the course of phonological development, children's error patterns decrease gradually. That is, the child does not continuously progress from 100% use of a certain error pattern to 0% use of that pattern. Progress in one area often starts and stops as other aspects of the child's language or phonology become the focus for some period of time.
- Error patterns that occur 40% or less of the time in the child's speech may continue to diminish without direct intervention.

Basic components of a process approach to intervention often include:
- Focus on one phonotactic and one phonetic error pattern at a time.
- Cycling through the child's error patterns, working on each for a set period of time before going on to focus on the next, regardless of the child's level of progress.
- Targeting error patterns that occur 40% or more of the time.
- The order in which processes are addressed in therapy may depend upon:
  —typical developmental order
  —effect on intelligibility
  —frequency of occurrence
  —stimulability

Alterations to the usual process approach to therapy that are appropriate for children with apraxia include:
- Pattern therapy is only one component of treatment.
- Typical developmental order is less likely to predict order of acquisition for children with apraxia; intelligibility and stimulability should be weighted more heavily.
- Regression and overgeneralization are common when related processes are targeted in close temporal proximity. Thus, it is better to avoid targeting similar processes (e.g., two different processes both affecting fricatives) close together.
- Apparent plateaus, during which no progress appears to be occurring, are not unusual. Changes that reflect the focus during such a cycle are often noticed at a later time. That is, there may be a delay in the effects of intervention.

INTONATION AND PROSODY: STRATEGIES FOR PRESCHOOL CHILDREN

- WHO? Preschool children with abnormal prosodic patterns.
- WHAT? A suggested set of goals for various aspects of prosody.
- WHY? Abnormal prosody strongly calls attention to itself, even if the speaker pronounces every segment correctly. Excess equal stress (a robot-like monostress/monopitch/monoloudness pattern) is a common characteristic of children with apraxia.
- LITERATURE RESOURCES: Davis & Velleman (2000); Velleman & K. Strand (1994, 1998); Velleman & Shriberg (1999).

Strategies for addressing intonation/prosody deficits among preschool children include the following.

Rhythm
- Drums, clapping, marching, and the like.
- Use to beat out number of syllables per word or to keep time with songs, rhymes, and so on.
- Provides rhythmic "frame" for word and syllable production.

Note: Beware of excess equal stress! Do not encourage robotic production, with each syllable equally stressed. Use big (loud, higher pitch) and small (quieter, lower pitch) drum or other toy to represent stressed versus unstressed syllables.

Pitch
- Animal sound keyboard: Imitate sound (chirp, bark, etc.) at "daddy" pitch (lowest note) versus "baby" (highest) versus "mommy" (middle) pitch.
- Songs, finger plays, and the like with varied pitch patterns.
- Play activities and books with animal voices, "daddy" versus "baby" voices, and so on.

Volume control
- Telling secrets, baby sleeping, and the like—whisper.
- BINGO, John Jacob Jingleheimer Schmidt, and other songs with loud and soft portions.
- "Wheels on the Bus" with loud versus soft voice for different verses (e.g., loud for "the baby on the bus says 'waah'"; soft for "the mommy on the bus says 'shhh'", etc.).

Duration/rate
- Songs sung at slow and fast rates.
- Finger plays at slow and fast rates.
- Walking and other gross motor games (e.g., "Lion Hunt") with longer duration words accompanying slower actions.

INTONATION AND PROSODY:
STRATEGIES FOR SCHOOL-AGE CHILDREN

- WHO? School-age children with abnormal prosodic patterns.
- WHAT? A suggested set of goals for various aspects of prosody.
- WHY? Abnormal prosody strongly calls attention to itself, even if the speaker pronounces every segment correctly. Excess equal stress (a robot-like, monostress pattern) is a common characteristic of children with apraxia. In some children, this stress pattern may be induced and then maintained by traditional apraxia therapy that emphasizes segmental accuracy at the cost of normal prosody. In others, it may be induced by reading-readiness syllable-counting activities that encourage children to produce multisyllabic words with excess equal stress. Alternatively, it may be an inherent characteristic of the disorder.
- LITERATURE RESOURCES: Velleman & K. Strand (1994, 1998); Velleman & Shriberg (1999); Wells & Peppé (in press).

Stress Patterns
- **Word Stress**: Have the child
    —Identify the number of syllables in a heard word (by clapping, with blocks, etc.).
    —Identify the stressed ("loud") syllable in orally presented multisyllabic words (e.g., represented by a larger block).
    —Imitate multisyllabic words with appropriate stress. (Use **backward build-ups** as needed to maintain appropriate prosody, including stress.)
    —Produce familiar (from steps 1–3) multisyllabic words with appropriate stress. (Use backward build-ups as needed to maintain appropriate prosody, including stress. Use different sizes of blocks as a visual cue for stressed versus unstressed syllables.)
- **Phrase Stress**:
    —Correctly match a spoken phrase with its meaning:

Example: black + board
with stress on "black," matches "what the teacher writes on"
with stress on "board," matches "a board that has been painted black."
Other examples include: white house, light house, green house, hot house, big top, fish tank, black bird, blue bird, hot dog.

    —Correctly stress a phrase to match the given meaning (production).

Sentence Stress:
- Identify the stressed ("loud") word in spoken sentences. (Stress may need to be exaggerated initially.)
- Given a wh-question, identify which word should be stressed in a written sentence. For example:

  "Who ate the cheese?" → "The *mouse* ate the cheese."
  "What did the mouse eat?" → "The mouse ate the *cheese*."
  "What did the mouse do to the cheese?" → "The mouse *ate* the cheese."

- Correctly acknowledge the correct response and repeat the sentence when modeled after marking the word to be stressed, for example, "Yes, the mouse *ate* the cheese."
- Given a wh-question, correctly stress the reply orally (as in the examples above).
- Given a written paragraph from a textbook, identify words that should be stressed (i.e., the most critical pieces of information) if the paragraph were to be read aloud.
- Given a written paragraph from a textbook, read it aloud after marking correct stress.
- Carry over these skills to:
  —Reading aloud in the classroom when forewarned of which portion of written text the child will be asked to read (so that she can independently pre-read it and select words to be stressed).
  —Appropriately stress words in controlled conversation (i.e., in therapy).
  —Appropriately stress words in conversation when asked to clarify an utterance (e.g., "Where did you go?" should be answered with stress on the location word).
Note: This is a very useful clarification strategy, as stressed words are louder and longer, and therefore clearer.
  —Appropriately stress words in spontaneous conversation.

Pitch (Sentence-Level)
- Identify rising pitch versus falling pitch at the ends of orally presented sentences:
  —In yes/no questions (rising) versus wh-questions and statements (falling pitch).
  —In lists (including counting)—rising pitch on all but last item, falling on last item. Signal when the last item is produced (based upon pitch cue).
- Given written sentences, indicate where the speaker should produce rising pitch versus falling pitch in the above environments.
- Given written sentences, orally produce rising pitch versus falling pitch in the above environments, first in imitation, then spontaneously.
- Given written paragraphs, mark words that should receive rising versus falling pitch, then read them aloud accordingly.
- Use pitch appropriately in controlled conversation (i.e., in therapy).
- Use pitch appropriately in conversation when asked to clarify an utterance.
- Use pitch appropriately in spontaneous conversation.

Pauses (**juncture**)

- Identify pauses within orally presented sentences.

  For example:
  —Between grammatical phrases:

  The big blue bird [pause] flew to the top of the tree.
  To the top of the tree [pause] the big blue bird [pause] flew.

  —Around adjectival phrases:

  That guy [pause] whom I told you about yesterday [pause] was there again today.

- Given written sentences, identify locations where pauses should occur (at edges of noun phrases, verb phrases, clauses, etc.).
- Repeat sentences with appropriate pauses (based upon prior identification).
- Read sentences with appropriate pauses (based upon prior identification).
- Use pauses appropriately in controlled conversation (i.e., in therapy).
- Use pauses appropriately in conversation when asked to clarify an utterance.
- Use pauses appropriately in spontaneous conversation.

INCREASING EARLY GRAMMATICAL
SKILLS IN CHILDREN WITH CAS

- WHO? Children with childhood apraxia who demonstrate concomitant delays/deficits in expressive language.
- WHAT? A suggested set of strategies specific to remediating language disorders in children with apraxia.
- WHY? Language deficits of particular sorts (see assessment section) often accompany childhood apraxia of speech.
- LITERATURE RESOURCES: Tyler (2002); Velleman & K. Strand (1994, 1998); Velleman & Shriberg (1999); Weiss (2001).

Specific strategies are suggested for language intervention with children with apraxia, including the following.

Do not speak **telegraphically!** To learn **function words** and morphology, the child must be exposed to them from the beginning. Therefore, do not say, for example, "Want toy?" Instead, say, "Do you want the toy?" You will automatically stress the words "want" and "toy," highlighting them for the child to imitate. The child may consciously ignore the function words, but will unconsciously learn from their presence and placement.

Stimulate use of early morphology by children with MLUs of at least 2.5 in the following order of ease of approximation:
- Early **free** (whole-word) **morphemes**: "in, on," and the like.
- "-ing".
- Irregular verb and noun forms that require:
  —salient vowel change (e.g., "mouse-mice," but *not* "woman-women"),
  —syllable addition (e.g., "child-children"), or
  —other change of greater than one phoneme (e.g., "think-thought").
- Syllabic forms of early bound morphemes, such as:
  —[əz] plural ("horses, boxes, houses, purses, couches, cheeses," etc.),
  —[əz] possessive ("Rose's, Mitch's," etc.),
  —[əz] third-person singular verb form ("kisses, matches, wishes," etc.),
  —[əd] past-tense verb form ("patted, padded, fitted, kidded, boated, loaded, weeded," etc.).
- Non-syllabic forms of early bound morphemes in vowel-final words, such as:
  —plural: "tubas, shoes"
  —possessive: "Rosa's, Joe's"
  —third-person singular verb form: "goes, fries"
  —past-tense verb form: "skied, tried," and so on.

Note: Remember that, like any child, the child with CAS may appear to learn irregular forms (such as "go"/"went") and then abandon them temporarily as regular forms are learned.

Improve sentence-building skills (for children with MLUs of 2.5 or better):
  • Address function words one by one, to 50% to 75% accuracy level.
  • Use visual or manual cues to mark sentence units.

> For example:
> —Blocks of different colors (with large ones to mark sentence stress) for different words.
> —Fokes Sentence Builder (Fokes, 1976) or other sequenced pictures to represent nouns, verbs, and adverbs.
> —Consistent gestures, objects, and the like to mark function words.

Use backward build-ups to maintain prosody in multisyllabic words and sentences

> For example:
> um
> ium
> quarium
> aquarium
> an aquarium
> in an aquarium
> lived in an aquarium
> turtle lived in an aquarium
> The turtle lived in an aquarium.

LITERACY

- WHO? Children with childhood apraxia who demonstrate concomitant delays/deficits in reading readiness and/or literacy, or who are at risk for such difficulties.
- WHAT? A suggested set of strategies specific to stimulating/remediating reading readiness and literacy skills in children with apraxia.
- WHY? Language deficits of particular sorts (see assessment section) often accompany childhood apraxia of speech.
- LITERATURE RESOURCES: Boynton (1984); Cunningham (1996); Gretz (1998); Hempenstall (1999); Lindamood & Lindamood (1998); Marion, Sussman, & Marquardt (1993); Martin (1996); Moreau & Fidrych-Puzzo (1994); Most (1996, 1997a,b); Pehrsson & Robinson (1985); Seuss (1996); Snowling & Stackhouse (1983); Stackhouse (1982, 1997); Stackhouse & Wells (1997, 2000); Stackhouse, Wells, Pascoe & Rees (2002).

Suggested order for increasing phonological awareness and skills:
- Linguistic units (illustrated in examples below):
  sentence level
  word level
  syllable level
  onset rhyme
  phoneme level
  The phoneme level is typically far more difficult for children than any of the others.
- Type of processing required (described in more detail below):
  recognizing relationships
  building part-whole relationships from given parts
  producing relationships (not all parts are given)
  breaking units down into smaller units.

Recognizing relationships: Give the child a set of two or more items (sentences, compound words, words, or syllables). Ask which ones have the same parts.

—Words in sentences (e.g., "Mary is sad," "Mary likes ice cream": Do the two sentences have anything the same in them?)

—Component words in compound words (e.g., "doghouse", "houseboat": Do the two words have anything the same in them?)

—Syllables/morphemes in words (e.g., "untie", "undo": Do the two words have anything the same in them?)

—Onset + rhyme in words/syllables (e.g., "cat", "hat" or "cat", "cup": Do the two words have anything the same in them?)

—Phonemes in syllables/words (e.g., "cat", "put": Do the two words have anything the same in them?)

Building part-whole relationships: Give the child the components, with small pauses between them, and ask him or her to give back the whole.

—Words in sentences (e.g., "Mary" + "is" + "sad" → "Mary is sad".)

Note: Use backward build-ups to help children produce sentences with natural intonation.

—Component words in compound words (e.g., "dog" + "house" → "dog-house")

—Syllables in words (e.g., "ba" + "na" + "na" → "banana")

Note: Use backward build-ups to help children pronounce words with natural intonation.

—Onset + rhyme in words/syllables (e.g., [k] + [æt] → "cat")

—Phonemes in syllables/words (e.g., [k] + [æ] + [t] → "cat")

Producing relationships: Give the child one item, and ask for another with the same component(s).

—Words in sentences (e.g., "Mary is sad": Make another sentence about "Mary," about "sad," etc.)

—Component words in compound words (e.g., "doghouse": Make another word with "house" in it, with "dog" in it, etc.)

—Syllables/morphemes in words (e.g., "untie": Make another word with "un" in it.)

—Onset + rhyme in words/syllables (e.g., "cat": Make another word that ends with "at" *and/or* Make a word that rhymes with "cat.")

—Phonemes in syllables/words (e.g., "cat": Make another word that starts with [k] (easiest); that ends with [t]; that has [æ] in it.)

Breaking down part-whole relationships: Give the child the whole, and ask him or her to give back one part, or the whole minus one part.

—Words in sentences (e.g., What's the first word in the sentence, "Mary is sad"?)

—Component words in compound words (e.g., Say "doghouse," but don't say "dog.")

—Syllables in words (e.g., Say "banana," but don't say "ba.")

—Phonemes in syllables/words (e.g., Say "cat," but don't say [k] (easiest); don't say [t].)

Note: It is much easier for children to do this task when it involves dividing the word into onset + rhyme, that is, removing the first consonant. Breaking up the rhyme, that is, removing the final consonant, is far more difficult.

Increase **phoneme-grapheme awareness** and skills
  • Visual recognition of similarities and differences among words (length, shape of printed word, inclusion of common elements).
  • Visual recognition of components of words (number of letters).
  • Recognition of specific letters by name ("This is the letter 't'.").
  • Recognition of specific letters by sound ("This letter makes the [t] sound.").
  • Recognition of common sight words (ability to read them aloud).
  • Recognition of common rhymes (e.g., "at," "op," "un," "ing": ability to read them).
  • Ability to blend
    —Two known words into a compound (e.g., "dog" + "house" → "dog-house").
    —Two known syllables or morphemes into one word (e.g., "go" + "ing" → "going").
    —Known onset + known rhyme into new syllable or word (e.g., "p" + "at" → "pat").
    —Individual phonemes into one syllable or word (e.g., "f" + "i" + "n" → "fin").
  • Recognition of digraph onsets (ability to read syllables or words that begin with "sh," "th," etc.: e.g. "ch" + "in" → "chin").
  • Recognition of non-phonetic rhymes (ability to read syllables or words that end with "igh," "ion," etc.: e.g. "s" + "igh").
  • Recognition of rhymes with multiple pronunciations (ability to read syllables or words that end with "ough," "ow," etc.).
  • Recognition that different rhymes may sometimes sound the same ("ough," "ow," etc.).

Informal strategies to increase reading readiness
  • Read **predictable book**s (e.g., Boynton, 1984; Martin, 1996).
  • Read rhyming books (e.g., Seuss, 1996).
  • Read books with puns or other wordplay (e.g., Most, 1996, 1997a,b).

SECTION

CASE STUDIES

....

TOPIC I: LIMITED WORD AND SYLLABLE STRUCTURES

Many children with CAS exhibit severe restrictions on the variety of word and syllable shapes that they can produce. These restrictions may be manifested by the production of very simple, universal syllable types such as open consonant vowel (CV) syllables. Other simplifications may be less in keeping with the tendencies of the languages of the world. For example, disyllables (two-syllable words) are more common universally than monosyllables, yet some children's phonotactic repertoires are limited to monosyllables. Consonant-alone and vowel-alone syllables are less common in the languages of the world than CV syllables, yet some children with CAS seem to have difficulty at the very basic level of combining a consonant with a vowel into a CV syllable. Some of these patterns are exemplified in the two children described below.

Case 1

Child: CW,[1] male
Age: 5;4
Background: At the time of this author's first evaluation of him, CW had been in therapy for two years. By report, at the age of 3 he had had no consonants in his repertoire. At 5 years of age, CW was doing well in kindergarten in all respects with the exception of expressive language (due to his severe phonological deficit).
Assessment results: CW's score on the Hodson (1986) *Assessment of Phonological Processes—Revised* at this time was 71, which fell in the profound range. His **percent consonants correct** (PCC; Shriberg & Kwiatkowski, 1982) was 79%. That is, in

words for which the target word could be identified, the consonants that he attempted were produced accurately 79% of the time (Shriberg, Aram, & Kwiatkowski, 1997c). However, many of his target words were quite uninterpretable, in utterances such as [dɪ mi ʌ] and [ʌ ʌ ʃp ʊm ʃp ʊm], despite accompanying gestures.

Phonotactic repertoire:
Syllable types:
- Open syllables were predominant: CV 60%; V 16%.
- Closed syllables were occasionally pronounced: VC 10%; CVC 18%.
- C alone occurred 3% of the time, including two productions of [ʃp]—two consonants in sequence with no vowel before, after, or between them.
- No clusters (with the possible exception of the two productions of [ʃp]).

Word shapes:
- Monosyllables predominant at 95%.
- Remaining 5% of words were disyllables.

Reduplication and harmony:
- 40% of two-syllable words (that is, two of the five) were reduplicated.
- 20% of two-syllable words (one of the five) included vowel harmony; none included consonant harmony.
- None of CW's CVC words included consonant harmony.

Phonetic repertoire: (phones that occurred at least three times in the sample; those that occurred, but less often, are in parentheses)

Initial consonants:

b	d	
m	n	(ŋ)
(w)	(j)	
(f)	(s)	(ʃ)*

Medial consonants:

(d)	(ʔ)
(n)	

Final consonants:

(b)		
p*	t	(k)
(m)	(n)	
	(s)	
	(tʃ)	

*produced twice in [#ʃp#]

Vowel repertoire:

i	(u)	
ɪ	(ʊ)	
	(o)	
ɛ		
æ	ʌ, ə	ɑ
aɪ, aʊ		

Analysis of results: CW's strengths included the ability to close syllables without using consonant harmony. Other positive factors included the emergence of a variety of vowels, consonants in initial position, and the ability to produce some two-syllable words, including some without reduplication or harmony. His weaknesses included a predominance of monosyllabic open-syllable words, resulting in very sparse consonant repertoires in medial and final positions. It was also noted that his spontaneous speech was rife with neutral vowel fillers, as in [ʌ ʌ ʌ fɪt mi] for "It didn't fit me." In addition, he omitted weak syllables, especially in initial position; for example, "Amanda" was pronounced as [mɪdʊ].

Intervention: Phonotactic goals, such as producing more two-syllable words and more closed syllables, were targeted until CW's ability to produce these structures improved. Reducing reduplication and harmony in two-syllable words was not addressed initially. Syllable repetition drills (using a "baba board," so-nicknamed by this child—see treatment section and glossary) were used to increase his motor-planning skills. He had particular difficulty maintaining distinct vowels in a series such as [ba bi bu bo baɪ], even when well-mastered consonants and vowels were used. Changes in consonant place of articulation, for well-mastered consonants, were not quite as difficult. As he learned to read, he used the printed words at the bottoms of the pictures to cue himself. As he became able to maintain alternating vowel or consonant places or manners of articulation, it became feasible to address the accuracy of his consonant productions, and to add specific phonetic targets (e.g., [f] in initial position).

Outcome: At 8;5, after three more years of intensive treatment, CW improved his score on the APP-R to 35, which falls in the moderate range. His PCC had not improved (in fact, his score was now very slightly down to 78% [as per Shriberg, Aram, & Kwiatkowski, 1997c]), because his speech was now intelligible enough that his target words could be identified more reliably and he was also attempting far more complicated word shapes and a much wider variety of sounds. Previously, the only words that he could produce intelligibly were very simple ones; unintelligible words are not used to compute PCC. Now, he was able to produce two-element clusters and multisyllabic words intelligibly—a feat that was not even a long-term goal at 5;4—but not without many sound substitutions. Therefore, it was now possible to determine exactly how inaccurate all of his productions were, and this had a negative effect on his PCC. At this point, the focus of his phonology therapy had shifted to the accurate production of specific sound classes (i.e., liquids) in particular positions (e.g., in clusters).

Case 2

Child: Holly, female (first reported in Velleman, 1994)

Age: 2;4

Background: No family history of speech, language, or learning difficulties. Holly babbled and began producing words at the expected ages (7–12 months; 12 months), but she vocalized/spoke infrequently. At 2;4, she was very shy and clingy, reluctant to be without her mother, who served as her translator.

Assessment results:

Phonotactic repertoire:
Syllable types:
- Open syllables were predominant: CV 48%; V 14%.
- Closed syllables were rare: CVC 5%.
- C alone (including tongue click) occurred 28% of the time.
- No clusters were produced.

Word shapes:
- Monosyllables were predominant at 95%.
- Remaining 5% of words were disyllables: VCV or CVCV.

Phonetic repertoire:
Consonants used in isolation (i.e., word is composed of a sole consonant):

t^h	39%
t^s	19%
click	16%
ʃ	10%
m	7%
Φ (voiceless bilabial fricative)	6%
n	3%

Consonants within syllables: (phones that occurred at least three times in the sample; those that occurred, but less often, are in parentheses)

Initial consonants:

b   d   (ʔ)
(m)   (n)
w

                        h

Medial consonants:

(b)
(m)
(w)   j   (h)
              (ʃ)

Final consonants:

                       ʔ
(m)
              (s)   h
          (ʒ)

Vowel repertoire:

i   (u)
ɪ   ʊ
e   o
ɛ   ɔ
(æ)   ʌ, ə   ɑ
    aɪ, aʊ

Analysis of results: Of particular concern was Holly's tendency to use a conso-nant alone to represent an entire word, such as [m] to represent food or the act of eat-ing. Solo alveolar consonants ([tʰ, tˢ]) and also an alveolar tongue click were used, apparently interchangeably, to represent a wide variety of nouns whose targets begin with non-labial consonants, including "tree," "coffee," and "kitty." Thus, the phrase "cat food" was often pronounced as [tˢ m:] (although this could also mean "kitty eat-ing," or "coffee is yummy," or a variety of other messages). Holly also used [d] + vari-ous (unpredictable) vowels to represent all deictics (this, that, there): [dɪ], [dɛ], [deɪ], [di], and [dɑ]. Nouns beginning with a target [b] or [p] (e.g., "bunny, bear, bird, baby, bell, pig, Bert") were pronounced very similarly, as [bɛə] or [bɪʊ]. As a result, there was a great deal of homonymy in her system. Other words were pronounced quite inconsistently. "Yes," for example, was produced variously as [daɪ], [dɛs], [hɑɪ], [aɪʃ], or [dɑɪʒ]; "no" as [nɑ] or [o]. These factors combined to make Holly very difficult to understand.

Intervention: Functional priorities for Holly were to decrease homonyms and variability in order to increase her intelligibility. Homonymy was decreased by expand-ing her word and syllable shapes to include more disyllables and CVC words (e.g., "bunny" as a two-syllable word versus "bear" as one syllable). Variability was decreased by targeting the consistency of word forms (e.g., feigning confusion when forms with [ɑɪ] were used to mean "yes"). As would be expected at her age, Holly was resistant to structured drill-like activities (e.g,. the baba board), so the same type of syllable rep-etition was practiced within play routines (e.g., saying "bowl bowl bowl" as [bo bo bo] while setting the table) and counting-book reading (e.g., saying "Three balls. Ball, ball, ball" rather than "one, two, three") instead. Her mother carried this approach over to home routines as well.

Outcome: Holly was very creative in her strategies for increasing her own com-municative effectiveness. As she became able to use whole-syllable forms (instead of solo consonants) for content words, she "recycled" her alveolar consonant/click pat-tern as fillers for function words (e.g., [bɑpɑ tʰ hiə] for "Papa's not here" and [tʰ dɪ do] for "Where this go?").

When Holly turned 3 years of age, her therapy was continued within the public school system. Unfortunately, the first year of therapy was devoted to a single goal: pro-duction of [f]. Although she made progress on that particular goal, her phonological sever-ity rating on the APP-R remained at the severe level. Consonant cluster reduction and final consonant deletion continued to be predominant phonotactic patterns. Fronting of velars, gliding as well as omission of liquids, and omission and stopping of stridents (with the exception of [f]) continued to be phonetic concerns. A cycles approach, with one pho-netic and one phonotactic goal addressed at a time, cycling every two to three months to another pair of goals, regardless of progress, was strongly recommended.

TOPIC II: CONSONANT-VOWEL DEPENDENCIES

Research (MacNeilage & Davis, 1990; Davis & MacNeilage, 1995) has shown that infants' babbles tend to be "homorganic." That is, babies have a strong tendency to produce syllables that require a minimum of tongue movement between the consonant and the vowel. Thus, alveolar consonants tend to co-occur with high front vowels ([didi, nɪnɪ], etc.), velars with high back vowels ([gugu], etc.), and labials with neutral and low vowels ([mʌmʌ, bɑbɑ], etc.). Although most adult languages persist in this tendency to a statistically significant extent, spoken words are not limited to these combinations, even in very young, normally developing children. However, some children with CAS appear to make minimal use of tongue mobility, especially intrasyllabically. Therefore, these limited consonant-vowel dependency patterns can sometimes be identified in children with CAS. An example is provided below.

Case 1

Child: Marina (first reported in Velleman, 1994)
Age: 3;11
Background: Marina began babbling at 12 months, and said her first word at 16 months. Her vocal progress was very slow; she was also delayed in gross and fine motor skills. She displayed oral, limb, and body apraxia as well as childhood apraxia of speech, with special difficulty sequencing movements of any kind. Marina's speech was slow and effortful, characterized by perseveration and struggle. Controlling oral secretions (drooling) was still an issue. Her receptive language, as well as her expressive language, was delayed and her attention span was quite short (indicating a more generalized delay or disorder, with apraxia as a secondary rather than as a primary diagnosis). In two-word utterances, a gesture often served in the place of one of the target spoken words.

Assessment results:

Phonotactic repertoire:
Syllable types:
• Open syllables were predominant: CV 72%.
• Closed syllables were occasionally produced: CVC 9%; VC 13%.
• Syllables consisting of a V produced alone or a C produced alone occurred 6% of the time (total).
• No clusters were observed.

Word shapes:
• CV monosyllables occurred 68% of the time; the remainder of words were disyllables.
• Harmonized consonants occurred in disyllables 64% of the time.
• Harmonized consonants occurred in monosyllables (CVC) 50% of the time.

Syllable-level effects (consonant-vowel affiliations):
• Labial consonants co-occurred with both high back and low back vowels 52% of the time, and co-occurred with mid vowels 38% of the time.
• Coronal (alveolar and palatal) consonants co-occurred with front vowels 48% of the time, with mid vowels 24% of the time, with low back vowels 20% of the time.

In short, labial consonants did not co-occur with front vowels, and coronal consonants rarely co-occurred with non-low back vowels.

Phonetic repertoire: (phones that occurred at least three times in the sample; those that occurred, but less often, are in parentheses)

Initial consonants:

b	d		
m	n		
w		(j)	
	(z)		
			tʃ

Medial consonants:

(b)	(d)		
(p)			
	(n)		
(w)		(j)	
		(tʃ)	

Final consonants:

	p			ʔ
(m)		n		
(f)		(s)	(ʃ)	

Vowels:

i		u
ɪ		(ʊ)
		o
(æ)	ʌ, ə	ɑ

Analysis of results: Of particular concern was Marina's tendency to use homorganic consonants and vowels within the same syllable (Davis & MacNeilage, 1995). That is, vowels requiring a raised front of the tongue (such as [i]) co-occurred with consonants of the same shape (e.g., [d]) but not with labial consonants, which do not require tongue raising. Thus, although Marina could say "daddy," she could not say "mommy" or "baby." She produced "baby" as either [didi] or [bɑbɑ], and called her mother "mom" rather than "mommy."

Intervention: A baba board was used with Marina to increase her ability to plan syllable productions. She used finger-pointing and torso-rocking to help establish the sequence and rhythm required for this activity, sometimes mis-sequencing with her finger and sometimes failing to vocalize in accompaniment to each rock. At first, she had great difficulty even repeating the same syllable more than twice in a row. Typically, the consonant or vowel deteriorated or the entire syllable was replaced by a grunt. The counting-like, prosodic contour of the syllable sequences seemed to be facilitative, and also carried over to an increase in two oral-word utterances. Apparently, this provided her with a rhythmic, melodic frame into which she inserted the target words. Backward build-ups were also very helpful in increasing her mean length of utterance, with very gradual carry-over from therapy into conversational speech.

Increasing the variety of consonant-vowel combinations that Marina could produce was also an early goal. Interestingly, it was in non-stressed final syllables that she first became able to produce labial consonant + high vowel combinations (e.g., "ba*by*"), in keeping with the final [i] pattern found in infant babbles and English child-directed speech ("dog*gie*", "hors*ie*", etc.; Davis & MacNeilage, 1995).

TOPIC III: STRONG FEATURE-BY-POSITION PATTERNS

Very young children (i.e., under the age of 30 months) who are normally developing sometimes evidence preferences for certain types of consonants to occur in certain word positions. It is not unusual, for example, for velars, nasals, and fricatives to be acquired first in final position, with other consonants acquired first in initial position. Some children even rearrange the consonants in the word (metathesis) in order to satisfy these preferences. (See Velleman, 1996 for a review.) Examples include a child nicknamed "W," who always moved fricatives to final position, as in [nupis] for "Snoopy" and even [aɪmf] for "fine" (Leonard & McGregor, 1991). Such patterns are typically short-lived, although they may be the source of significant confusion until they either disappear or the child's significant others figure out how to interpret affected words. In some cases, especially in children with CAS, such a pattern interferes enough with the child's intelligibility to warrant speech-language intervention. This was the case with "Ellen," described below.

Case 1

Child: Ellen (first reported in Velleman, 1998)
Age: 2;3
Background: Ellen was the second child of a speech-language pathologist whose son had been diagnosed with childhood apraxia of speech. As her vocabulary and mean length of utterance began increasing in her third year of life, Ellen's speech had become increasingly unintelligible. Both she and her family were quite frustrated in their attempts to communicate with each other.

Assessment results:

Phonotactic repertoire:
Syllable types:
- Open syllables were predominant: CV occurred 66% of the time; V alone occurred 21% of the time.
- Closed syllables were rarely produced: CVC occurred 10% of the time; VC occurred 2% of the time.

Word shapes:
- Monosyllables represented 50% of the words produced; disyllables represented 33%.
- Disyllables were reduplicated 38% of the time; consonant harmony occurred in disyllables 31% of the time.
- Consonant harmony occurred in CVC words 71% of the time.

Phonetic repertoire: (phones that occurred at least three times in the sample; those that occurred, but less often, are in parentheses)

Initial consonants:

b	d		(g)
p	t		
(m)	(n)		
w		(j)	
			(h)
	(dʒ)		

Medial consonants:

b	d		(ʔ)
(p)	(t)	(k)	
m	n		
w			
(v)			
(ɸ)			(h)

Final consonants:

	(d)	(g)
p	(t)	(k)

Vowels:

i		u
ɪ		ʊ
e		o
ɛ		ɔ
æ	ʌ, ə	ɑ
	aɪ, aʊ	

Analysis of results: Of particular concern in Ellen's case was her frequent use of consonant harmony, especially when it was discovered that consonant harmony and even reduplication were being applied at the phrase level as well. For example, Ellen produced "not in" as [ĩ ĩn], and "not bottle" as [ba baba]. These utterances were accompanied by a head shake "no" and other gestures, making their meanings clear. Thus, the same word (e.g., "no") was modified to match the other word in each utterance. When her unintelligible utterances were analyzed, it was noted that those utterances that did not demonstrate reduplication or consonant harmony demonstrated another pattern: labial C-V-alveolar C-V, often transcribed as [bʌdɪ]. Certain words that had been guessed from context also showed this same pattern: "kitty" ([bʌdə]), "panda" ([badə]), "blow it" ([bʌdɪʔ]), and "patty-cake" ([pæpita]. These patterns distorted her output to the extent that she was quite unintelligible, even (increasingly) to her mother, who was a pediatric speech-language pathologist herself.

Also of concern were her relatively infrequent use of final consonants and her frequent vowel deviations.

Intervention: The primary initial goal for Ellen was to increase the number of words that she produced with other patterns. First, CVCV words with two different consonants in a labial-alveolar pattern were targeted (to decrease harmony). Next, CVCV words with other consonant patterns (e.g., alveolar-labial) were targeted. An increase in CVC words produced with a final consonant was the next goal, with the first objective being CVC words with harmony, then CVC words with labial-alveolar patterns, then CVC words with other patterns. Phonetically, goals included accurate production of vowels and increasing use of emerging consonants (nasals in final position, velars and fricatives in any position).

Outcome: Ellen was reevaluated at the age of 4;0. Reduplication and harmony were rare. Closed syllables and even consonant clusters were common. She was producing a wide variety of consonants in a wide variety of positions. Yet, she had once again become quite unintelligible. Why? Phonetic analysis revealed that she had a very complex, apparently unpredictable pattern of substitutions for fricatives. Sometimes one fricative was substituted for another, but on other occasions velar stops, glides, and other consonants replaced fricatives. At this time, Ellen's old tendency toward harmony was used as a preliminary strategy for improving the accuracy of her fricative productions. That is, words with harmonizing fricatives (such as "shush" and "fluffy") were early targets.

TOPIC IV: PROSODIC ABNORMALITIES

Prosodic abnormalities are often cited as a symptom of CAS. In particular, Shriberg, Aram and Kwiatkowski (1997c) have posited excess equal stress—that is, monostress speech—as a hallmark of the disorder. In this author's clinical experience, some children with CAS who have relatively normal prosody with unintelligible speech seem to discover, possibly through therapy or preliteracy activities (e.g., counting syllables), that they are more intelligible if they speak slowly and haltingly, one word or syllable at a time. Others have no history of normal prosody. BL fits into the former category.

Case 1

Child: BL

Tested at ages: 6;3, 7;1, 8;6

Background information: BL had a history of hypotonia, motor-planning difficulties, and a receptive-expressive language gap. At the age of 6, he was still only 50% to 65% intelligible to this author in conversational speech. His attempts at syllable repetition and diadochokinesis were slow, effortful, and arrhythmic. He was making good progress toward his phonotactic goal of producing words with a front-to-back consonant pattern (e.g., labial-alveolar or labial-velar). However, he was beginning to demonstrate difficulties with early literacy skills.

Assessment results:

6;3: On the APP-R, BL scored at the severe level. Frequent phonotactic processes included consonant cluster reduction (75%) and final consonant deletion (32%). Several deviant processes were also noted, including fronting in initial and medial positions and backing (sometimes to uvular or pharyngeal places of articulation) in final position. It was felt that these patterns might result from overgeneralization of the front-to-back patterns that he had been practicing in therapy. Vowel deviations and voicing errors were also common. His speech was typically fluent (i.e., smooth and prosodically appropriate), but quite unintelligible.

7;1: 10 months later, BL's consonant cluster reduction had reduced slightly (to 70%), final consonant deletion even more (to 35%). He was more intelligible, but it was noted with some concern that his speech was becoming choppy, monotone, and monostress when he focused on accuracy.

8;6: When he was 8½, BL's lexical stress patterns were explicitly evaluated. He was observed to use weak syllable deletion in the same iambic contexts as those found in very young children who are normally developing and in children with childhood apraxia of speech (as described by Velleman & Shriberg, 1999). These results are given below. (*Note:* "W" stands for a weak, unstressed syllable; "S" represents a strong, stressed syllable.)

Syllable type omitted	Example
Initial W of WSW	[nɑsəwɪs] for "*rhi*noceros", [næenə] for "*ba*nana"
Initial W of WSWW	[spʌwɪgɪs] for "*a*sparagus"
Medial W of SWS	[bætʃɪs] for "pack*a*ges", [kæŋgwu] for "kang*a*roo"
1st medial W of SWSW	[bæklinʊ] for "va*cuum* cleaner"

BL also occasionally strengthened the vowels of initial weak syllables (weak syllable augmentation) or added an entire syllable, as in [bɪ́ketʃɪn] for "vacation" and [ðebʌrɛriən] for "librarian." Especially of concern was the fact that, as he became aware that the task was to produce multisyllabic words, BL began to count out the syllables by tapping on his arm. As he did so, his productions became even more monotone, monostress, and generally robotic. His use of this strategy increased his intelligibility markedly, but made his speech sound very odd and almost non-human.

Similar difficulties were noted when BL read aloud. He appeared to have no concept of how long a particular word should be, sometimes guessing a very short, familiar word in place of a longer one. He also showed no attempt to group sentence components appropriately. Each word was read with equal stress in a monotone. It was hypothesized that this might be affecting his reading comprehension as well as his intelligibility while reading aloud.

Intervention: Diagnostic therapy revealed that BL was able to identify the most stressed syllable of a word (e.g., "spa*ghet*ti") when it was produced by this author, but not when he produced it himself. He was not using contrastive sentence stress (e.g., "I want the *big* red one" versus "I want the big *red* one") either receptively or expressively. It was suggested that intervention focus explicitly on receptive and expressive use of stress patterns and other aspects of prosody, including preparsing of a sentence to identify and mark words that should be stressed and where pauses should fall, before he read it aloud.

---

[1] *Note:* This author's recordings of CW's speech at 5;4 and 8;5 were transcribed and analyzed as part of the study reported by Shriberg, Aram, & Kwiatkowski (1997c).

APPENDIX

ELECTRONIC RESOURCES

INFORMATION RESOURCES

Afasic. (2001). Developmental verbal dyspraxia: Information for parents from Afasic. Available 12/19/01 at http://www.apraxia-kids.org/faqs/afasic.html.

Afasic—Overcoming Speech Impairments, U.K. Web site: http://www.afasic.org.uk.

American Speech-Language Hearing Association Web site: http://www.asha.org/.

Apraxia Guide to Helpful Links and Resources: http://home.talkcity.com/SupportSt/lynettep1/index.html.

Apraxia-Kids Web site: http://www.apraxia.org/.

Apraxia of Speech Citations Web site: http://www.faughnan.com/apraxiarefs.html.

Childhood Apraxia of Speech Association Web site: http://www.apraxia.org.

Children's Apraxia Network/CHERAB Foundation Web site: http://www.apraxia.cc

Dyspraxia Foundation, U.K. Web site: http://www.emmbrook.demon.co.uk/dysprax/homepage.htm.

Gretz, S. (1998). Literacy development & children with apraxia of speech. Available 3/01 at http://www.apraxia-kids.org/literacy/literacy.html.

Guild, Ann S., & Vail, Tracy. (1999). Developmental verbal apraxia or developmental apraxia of speech. Available 12/19/01 at http://tayloredmktg.com/dyspraxia/das.html.

Hammer, D., & Stoeckel, R. (2001). Teaching and talking together: Building a treatment team. Available 12/19/01 at http://www.apraxia-kids.org/indexes/asha2001presentation.ppt.

The Hanen Centre—Helping Children Communicate Web site: http://www.hanen.org/.

Hempenstall, K. (1999). Beginning reading instruction: The role of phonemic awareness and phonics. *1999 Successful Learning Conference.* University of Western Sydney. Available 3/01 at http://www.rmit.edu.au/departments/ps/staffpgs/hempenart/1999.htm.

Lindamood-Bell Learning Processes Web site: http://lindamoodbell.com/.

Morris, S. E. (1997a). Feeding and speech relationships. Available 2/24/01 at http://www.new-vis.com/fym/papers/p-feed8.htm.

Morris, S. E. (1997b). Mouth toys open the sensory doorway. Available 2/24/01 at http://www.new-vis.com/fym/papers/p-feed1.htm.

Morris, S. E. (1997c). Stuffing. Available 2/24/01 at http://www.new-vis.com/fym/papers/p-feed11.htm.

Picture Exchange Communication System Web site: http://www.pecs.com/.

Prompt Institute Web site: http://www.promptinstitute.com/index2.html.

Vail, T. (2001). Treating apraxia in children with autism. Available 12/19/01 at http://www.apraxia-kids.org/slps/vail.html.

LISTSERVS AND SUPPORT GROUPS

Apraxia-Kids Listserv available at http://www.apraxia-kids.org/talk/subscribe.html.

Expressive Communication Help Organization (Ontario, Canada) Listserv: http://groups.yahoo.com/group/apraxiaontario/join.

How to start an apraxia support group available at http://home.talkcity.com/SupportSt/lynettep1/supportgroup.html.

Late Talkers Internet Parent Group available at http://groups.yahoo.com/group/Latetalkers/.

Parent Networks and Support Groups available at http://www.apraxia-kids.org/talk/support.html.

Phonological Disorders Listserv available at http://groups.yahoo.com/group/ phonod/.

SOFTWARE FOR SPEECH-LANGUAGE PATHOLOGISTS

Hodson, B. (1985). Computerized Assessment of Phonological Processes: Version 1.0 [Apple II series computer program]. Interstate: Danville.

Long, S., & Fey, M. (1993). Computerized Profiling: Version 1.0—Macintosh. San Antonio, TX: The Psychological Corporation.

Long, S., & Fey, M. (1993). Computerized Profiling: Version 7.0—DOS. San Antonio, TX: The Psychological Corporation.

Masterson, J., & Bernhardt, B. (2001). CAPES: Computerized Articulation and Phonology Evaluation System. San Antonio, TX: The Psychological Corporation.

Masterson, J., & Pagan, F. (1993). Interactive System for Phonological Analysis. San Antonio, TX: The Psychological Corporation.

Oller, K., & Delgado, R. (1990). Logical International Phonetic Programs (LIPP) Version 1.03. Miami, FL: Intelligent Hearing Systems.

Shriberg, L. (1986). Program to Examine Phonetic and Phonologic Evaluation Records, Version 4.0 (PEPPER). Hillsdale, NJ: Lawrence Erlbaum Associates.

Weiner, F. (1993, 1995). Automatic Articulation Analysis Plus [Windows computer program]. State College, PA: Parrot Software.

APPENDIX

SUGGESTED BOOKS FOR YOUNG CHILDREN WITH CAS

Boynton, S. (1984). *Blue hat, green hat.* New York: Simon & Schuster.

——. (1995). *Doggies.* New York: Simon & Schuster.

——. (1995). *Moo, baa, lalala.* New York: Simon & Schuster.

Chancellor D. (1999).*Copycat animals.* New York: DK Publishing.

——. (1999). *Copycat faces.* New York: DK Publishing.

Hill, E. (1980). *Where's Spot?* New York: Putnam.

Martin, B. (1996). *Brown bear, brown bear, what do you see?* New York: Henry Holt & Co.

Mayer, M. (1983). *I was so mad.* New York: Golden Books.

McGrath, B. B. (1994). *The m&m's counting book.* Watertown, MA: Charlesbridge.

Most, B. (1996). *Cock-a-doodle-moo!* New York: Harcourt Brace & Co.

————. (1997). *Moo ha.* New York: Harcourt Brace & Co.

————. (1997). *Oink ha.* New York: Harcourt Brace & Co.

Seuss, D. (1996). *There's a wocket in my pocket.* New York: Random House.

Wade, L. (1998). *The Cheerios®* animals play book. New York: Simon & Schuster.

————. (1998). The Cheerios® play book. New York: Simon & Schuster.

Zimmerman, R. (1996). *Ba ba ha ha.* Scarborough, ON: Harpercollins/Robert Zimmerman.

————. (1996). *Oooh oooh moo.* Scarborough, ON: Harper Collins/Robert Zimmerman.

APPENDIX

INTERNATIONAL PHONETIC ASSOCIATION SYMBOLS USED IN THIS BOOK

Shown in Table A-1 are orthographic symbols corresponding to the IPA symbols used in this book, and words to illustrate the corresponding sounds. The table does not include symbols for consonants that represent the same sound as the corresponding English letters: [p], [b], [t], [d], [k], [m], [n], [f], [v], [s], [z], [l], [w]. Note that some letters represent two or more sounds in English spelling (e.g., the letter "g" represents [g] in "go," [dʒ] in "George," and [ʒ] in "rouge"), and some sounds in English can be represented by more than one letter (e.g., the [s] sound can be spelled with "s", "c", or even sometimes "z"). In IPA, on the other hand, there is always a one-to-one symbol-to-sound correspondence. For further information consult the International Phonetic Association's Handbook (International Phonetic Association, 1999) or Web site (http://www2.arts.gla.ac.uk/IPA/ipa.html).

Table A-1. Orthographic Symbols, IPA Symbols, and Key Words

Consonants

Orthographic Symbol	IPA Symbol	Key Word
g	g	go
ng	ŋ	ring
y	j	you
r	ɹ	red
th	θ	thigh
th	ð	thy
sh	ʃ	shoe
g	ʒ	rouge
ch	tʃ	church
j, g	dʒ	judge
(glottal stop)	ʔ	uh-oh
(voiceless bilabial fricative)	ɸ	(does not occur in English)

Vowels

Orthographic Symbol	IPA Symbol	Key Word
ee, ea, ie, y	i	seed
i	ɪ	sit
a, ay, ai, a_e, ey	e	say
e	ɛ	said
a	æ	sad
u, ue, oo, u_e, ew	u	sue
oo	ʊ	soot
o, oa, o_e, ough, ow	o	soak
aw, au, augh, ough	ɔ	slaw
o	ɑ	stop
u	ʌ	supper
any vowel	ə	about
ir, ur	ɝ	sturdy
er	ɚ	sputter
ow, ough, au, ou	aʊ	spout
i, i_e, y, uy, igh	aɪ	sigh
oi, oy	ɔɪ	soy

Note: When stressed, [e] is sometimes pronounced as [eɪ], and [o] as [oʊ]. A blank line between two vowels indicates a consonant slot in English spelling. (E.g., "a_e" could be filled in with "t" as in "late," "p" as in "tape," "n" as in "mane," "c" as in "face," etc.).

GLOSSARY

· ·

Adult-onset apraxia of speech (AOS): A communication disorder that may result from a stroke or other neurological insult. *See also* Apraxia, Dyspraxia.

Affrication: Production of a speech sound (usually a stop or fricative) that normally has only one manner of articulation as a sequence of two places of articulation. Examples: [ʃ] or [t] pronounced as [tʃ]; [z] or [d] pronounced as [dz].

Alliteration: "Repetition of the same consonant, especially an initial one, in several words within the same sentence or phrase" (Nicolosi, Harryman, & Kresheck, 1996, p. 6). Example: "Lisa's lovely lilies languished on the lawn."

Alternating repetitive motion (ARM): Alternating repetition of the same movement or syllable (e.g., [pʌtʌpʌtʌpʌtʌ]). Also called "diadochokinesis."

Apraxia: "A disorder in carrying out or learning complex movements that cannot be accounted for by elementary disturbances of strength, coordination, sensation, comprehension, or attention" (Strub & Black, 1981, p. 232). *See* adult-onset apraxia, childhood apraxia, developmental dyspraxia, dyspraxia.

Automatic speech: Phrases, sentences, or longer stretches of discourse that are so well learned that no motor planning is required; an existing motor plan can be recruited. Examples: social niceties, pledge of allegiance, prayers, children's songs, alphabet, counting, Christmas carols.

Baba board: A set of flip books designed to facilitate syllable practice activities, constructed as follows. Paste the same set of pictures representing the target syllables into several 3 x 5 spiral notebooks. Then, line the notebooks up on the table (or hang them over a hanging file drawer frame), flipping pages as appropriate. Group pictures phonetically. For example, the first section of each stops book includes syllables with initial [b]: bee, baa, boo, bow, boy, buy, bay. Thus, the entire row of stops books could be lined up and turned to the "bee" page, for the child to point to and name one by one. The next section in the stops book could be [d] syllables, in the same sequence of vowels (as possible, given that some syllables will not be picturable): dee, (no picture for [da]), dew, doe/dough, day. The voiceless stops sections (usually at the end of the stops book, as initial voiceless stops are more difficult than initial voiced stops) would include [p] with: pea, pa, Pooh, pie, pay, paw, pow; and so on. Other sets of books would include glide-initial syllables, fricative-initial syllables, and so on. Mayer-Johnson pictures may be useful for this purpose. For older children who have some literacy skills, syllables can be written out instead. Be careful to spell the syllables/words not in IPA but as they would be spelled in English orthography!

Backing: Production of a speech sound farther back in the oral cavity than is usual (for either articulatory or phonological reasons). Typically refers to production of alveolar sounds (e.g., [t]) in velar position (i.e., as [k]).

Backward build-up: Practice (e.g., modeling followed by imitation) of a multisyllabic word, phrase, or sentence from the end to the beginning, in ever-larger chunks, to preserve normal intonation contours. Example:

bumpers

buggy bumpers

baby buggy bumpers

rubber baby buggy bumpers

Blending: Fluent production of the sounds in a written word, spoken as a word. Example: C-A-T pronounced as "cat."

Bound morpheme: Morpheme that only occurs in conjunction with another morpheme. Example: "nym" has no meaning on its own, but must be combined with "anto-", "homo-", "syno-", "pseudo-", or some other morpheme.

Canonical babble: Infants' production of meaningless, repetitive syllables with alternating "true" consonants (neither glottals nor glides) and full vowels.

Carrier phrase: A phrase or sentence in which one word or phrase may vary, typically in the final position. Example: "Let's go _____," where the blank could be filled with "play," "eat," "climb a tree," and so forth.

CAS: Childhood apraxia of speech.

Centralization of vowels: Production of front or back vowels more centrally (in the middle of the mouth). Example: production of [i] or [ɑ] as [ʌ].

Childhood apraxia of speech (CAS): A type of apraxia/dyspraxia that appears to be congenital. That is, it is present from birth (although it may not be identified until later), and no neurological insult or other cause is known. Also referred to as developmental verbal dyspraxia (DVD), developmental apraxia of speech (DAS), and other terms. In this book, the term "childhood apraxia of speech" is used.

Chronological mismatch: A situation in which some of a child's skills (e.g., phonological processes) are delayed to a greater extent than other skills (e.g., phonetic repertoire).

Coda: The final consonant or cluster of a syllable.

Combinatorial play: Ability to construct a whole from parts or to recognize parts of a whole in play (e.g., stacking nesting cups).

Communicative intent: The meaning that the speaker is trying to convey.

Communicative means: The modality that the speaker uses to convey his or her meaning (e.g., words, gestures, facial expressions, etc.).

Compound word: A word composed of two or more free morphemes (words), such as "birdhouse", "mailbox", and the like.

Consonant cluster coalescence: The merger of two consonants in a cluster into one, based upon the features of each. For example, borrowing the frication (continuance) of the [s] and the labiality of the [w] in "swing" would yield [fɪŋ]: [f] is a labial (like [w]) fricative (like [s]).

Constraint: A phonological/linguistic restriction that prevents the occurrence of a particular output in a person's speech or in a particular language. Example: A child with a constraint against velars would avoid producing these sounds (via omission, fronting, etc.).

Corner vowels: *See* Vowel triangle.

Deaffrication: Production of an affricate (in English, [tʃ] or [dʒ]) as a simple consonant (e.g., [t] or [ʃ], [d] or [ʒ]).

Denasalization: Production of a nasal target consonant without nasality.

Desensitization: A decrease in a person's reactivity to a certain stimulus. Example: A person who has not been fed orally may have a strong negative reaction to food flavors. Tiny, diluted tastes may be put on her or his tongue to gradually decrease these negative reactions.

Developmental apraxia of speech (DAS): *See* Childhood apraxia.

Developmental verbal dyspraxia (DVD): *See* Childhood apraxia.

Deviant process: A phonological pattern, such as initial consonant deletion, that does not occur in children who are normally developing.

Devoicing: Production of a voiced sound (e.g., [b]) without voicing (e.g., as [p]).

Diadochokinesis (DDK): *See* Alternating repetitive motion.

Distributed practice: Repetition of many targets sharing a common gestural basis (e.g., a series of words beginning with the [θ] sound).

Dysarthria: "A group of motor speech disorders resulting from disturbed muscular control of the speech mechanism due to damage of the peripheral or central nervous system; oral communication problems due to weakness, incoordination, or paralysis of speech musculature; physiologic characteristics often include abnormal or disturbed strength, speed, range, steadiness, tone, and accuracy of muscle movements" (Hegde, 1996, p. 180).

Dysphagia: Difficulty swallowing due to physical disease, damage, or disorder.

Dyspraxia: Technically refers to a mild apraxia. In practice, the terms "apraxia" and "dyspraxia" are often used interchangeably.

Embedded play routine: Play routine having a plot or a theme, with interrelated levels, types, or sequences of actions.

Epenthesis: Insertion of an extra consonant or vowel within a syllable or word (e.g., "blue" pronounced as [bəlu]). Often changes the structure of the word, for example, by adding an extra syllable and/or separating the elements of a cluster.

Excess equal stress: A pattern of monostressed syllables and words that makes a child's speech sound very robotic (Shriberg, Aram & Kwiatkowski 1997a, b, c).

Executive apraxia: A form of apraxia characterized by highly motoric symptoms (such as groping and articulatory errors that occur even in simple syllables or words) (Crary 1993).

Failure to thrive: A life-threatening disorder of infancy, in which the infant does not grow or progress at a normal rate; may have physiological, psychological, social, or other causes.

Feet: Units of prosody or rhythm, as in poetry. The typical foot in English includes two syllables.

Frame: The structure of a word or sentence. In phonology, the phonotactics (word and syllable shapes, such as CCVCVCC or a strong-weak-strong-weak stress pattern) serve as the frame, and the phonetic elements (specific consonant and vowel features) provide the content that is inserted into the frame.

Free morpheme: A morpheme that can stand on its own. Many free morphemes can also be combined with other morphemes, but they are grammatical and make sense alone as well (e.g., "berry" can be combined with "blue" or "straw" or "boysen-", but it has meaning and grammatical function alone).

Frication: The production of a phoneme from some other manner of articulation class as a fricative. Considered to be a deviant process: that is, children who are typically developing rarely exhibit this pattern.

Fronting: Production of a target phoneme in a place of articulation that is farther front than in the target. Typically applies when a velar is pronounced as alveolar (e.g., "cake" as [teɪt]).

Function word: A word that serves a grammatical function only, such as a preposition or an article. Function (or closed class) words belong to a much smaller set than content words (e.g., there are a limited number of articles in English, but no limit to the number of nouns).

Grading of movements: Modulation of the force or extent of a movement as appropriate to the physical task at hand. Poor movement grading may result in overshoot or undershoot (see definitions).

Harmony: Production of two (or more) consonant or vowel sounds in a way that makes them the same or at least more similar than in the target, resulting in a word that is easier to pronounce. Example: "doggie" pronounced as [dɔdi] or [gɔgi] (consonant harmony) or as [digi] or [dɔgɔ] (vowel harmony). Also called "assimilation."

Hierarchy: A ranking of elements on different levels (such as the hierarchy of administrators in a business).

Homonym: A word that sounds the same as another, but has a different meaning. Example: "right", "write", and "rite".

Homorganic: Produced at the same place or in the same manner of articulation. Example: "in" becomes "im" to form the word "impossible": [m] and [p] are homorganic. High front vowels have a statistical tendency to co-occur with syllables that have alveolar onsets. In the syllable [di]: [d] and [i] are homorganic.

Hypersensitivity: More than the usual level of responsivity to a stimulus; a low threshold of reactivity. Example: People who get car sick are hypersensitive to movements of certain types.

Hyposensitivity: Less than the usual level of responsivity to a stimulus; a high threshold of reactivity. Example: A person who always keeps the television on in the background becomes hyposensitive to the sound of it.

Ideomotor apraxia: An inability to conceptualize a novel motor plan.

Initial consonant deletion: Failure to produce the target onset consonant of a word. Example: "book" pronounced as [ʊk]. Considered a deviant phonological process (not expected in the normal course of phonological development) in children learning English.

Intrusive schwa: A schwa (unstressed neutral vowel) that is epenthesized, that is, pronounced in a position in which the sound does not normally occur in the target word; most commonly occurs between two consonants within a cluster. Example: "blue" pronounced as [bəlu].

Jargon: A form of prelinguistic vocal behavior in which a variety of consonants and vowels are produced with sentencelike intonation contours and rhythm. Some Anglo American parents refer to this as "telling stories" or "speaking Chinese" because it sounds as if the child is speaking in sentences that are not intelligible.

Juncture: A pause, decrease in pitch, or other phonetic feature that occurs at a grammatical boundary in a phrase or sentence.

Mass practice: In therapy, many repetitions of a small number of target sounds, syllables, or words.

Mean Babbling Level (MBL): A formula, based upon type and variety of consonants produced, for calculating the maturity of a child's prelinguistic vocalizations.

Melodic Intonation Therapy (MIT): The use of rhythms or pitch patterns to facilitate speech production.

Metalinguistic awareness: The ability to consciously reflect upon and/or talk about language.

Metathesis: The interchange of two speech sounds within a word or phrase. More common in developing and disordered phonologies than in adult languages. Examples: Modern English "ask" was "acsian" in Old English; this author's first phonology client (a 4-year-old) pronounced "bug" as [gʌb].

Migration: The movement of a speech sound to a non-target position in a word. Example: "snack" pronounced as [næks].

Monoloud: Produced without variations in loudness.

Monopitch: Produced without variations in pitch.

Monostress: Produced without variations in stress.

Morpheme: The smallest unit of meaning in a language; may stand alone (free morpheme) or occur only in conjunction with others (bound morpheme). Examples of bound morphemes in English include: "dis-", "re-", "-ing", "-ed", "-able", "-ette".

Multimodal inputs: Stimulation to a variety of sensory systems (e.g., visual, auditory, tactile, etc.) at once.

Munch: A combined sucking-biting-chewing motion, usually in the anterior portion of the mouth; typically seen before mature chewing patterns are established. The tongue and jaw may go up and down, but the tongue does not move to the sides to propel the food between the teeth.

Muscle tone: "The resting level of tension in a muscle; in general, it prepares the muscle for a rapid and reliable response to voluntary or reflexive commands" (Purves et al., 1997, p. 305).

Nasal resonance: Nasality resulting from vibrations in the nasal cavity. Considered to be normal when co-occurring with nasal consonants (e.g., in the phrase "ninety-nine"), but not with oral consonants (e.g., in the phrase "eighty-eight").

Nasalization: Production of a non-nasal speech sound as nasal. Example: "dad" pronounced as [næn].

Non-speech communication: Means of communication that do not depend on oral speech production, such as sign, gesture, writing, and the like.

Nucleus: The part of the syllable that carries the pitch and loudness, usually a vowel or diphthong.

Onset: The initial consonant or consonant cluster of a syllable or word.

Oral-motor reflex: An involuntary motor response to stimulation of the oral motor area. Example: Infants open their mouths and turn toward a touch to the cheek—the rooting reflex.

Overflow: Movement of a part of the body that affects nearby structures more than intended.

Overshoot: Movement of a part of the body that is extended to more of a degree than was intended or is appropriate for accurate articulation.

Percent Consonants Correct: A method for calculating intelligibility based upon the proportion of the consonants that a person attempts to produce which are produced correctly (Shriberg & Kwiatkowski, 1982). For example, if the word "string" (/stɹɪŋ/) is pronounced as [stwɪŋ], three of the four consonants were pronounced correctly, for a PCC of 75%.

Phonatory control: Control of phonation, that is, the vibration of the vocal cords.

Phonetic repertoire: The set of consonants and vowels used by a particular speaker or in a certain language.

Phoneme: The smallest unit of sound that provides contrast within a language. Example: /p/ and /b/ are different phonemes in English, because they cannot be interchanged without changing the meaning of the word (e.g., "bat" and "pat," "lab" and "lap," are different words with contrastive meanings).

Phoneme/grapheme awareness: Knowledge of the relationship between letters and sounds. Example: The letter *b* represents the sound [b]. Also called "sound-letter correspondence."

Phonological patterns: Consistent errors affecting entire classes of structures (e.g., all final consonants are deleted) or entire classes of sounds (e.g., all fricatives are pronounced as stops). Includes processes and constraints.

Phonotactic repertoire: Syllable and word shapes.

Phrase stress: Stress (in English, the combination of increased loudness, duration, and pitch) used to identify the relationship between words within a phrase (e.g., "the white *house*" is a house that is white; "the *white* house" is where the president lives).

Planning apraxia: "Difficulty with longer, more complex sequences of speech and oral motor behavior . . . difficulty with selection and ordering of targets within a sequence." (Crary, 1993, pp. 60–61).

Praxis: The ability to conceive of, prepare, and initiate a volitional motor pattern.

Precanonical babble: Rhythmic babble in which the consonants are glottal stops, nasals, glides, or prolonged resonants/fricatives. Timing and extent of opening (for vowels) and closing (for consonants) are not yet adultlike.

Predictable book: Book in which the plot, and therefore the wording, is repetitious, thus making it easier for the reader to predict what words or events will come next. Examples: "Where's Spot?" (Hill, 1980); "I was so mad" (Mayer, 1983), "Blue hat, green hat" (Boynton, 1984).

Pretend play/symbolic play: Ability to use one object to represent another. At a higher level, ability to use an imagined object to represent a real object.

Phonological process: A type of phonological pattern whose label refers to the change made in the target word. Example: Pronouncing "fish" as [pɪʃ] is an example of stopping because the fricative [f] is pronounced as a stop, [p].

Prosody: A phonological feature that spreads over more than one word. Includes tone, pitch, and stress (which itself includes, in English, higher pitch and intensity, and longer duration).

Receptive-expressive language gap: A situation in which a person's receptive language is significantly better than his or her expressive language; typically, receptive language is within normal limits.

Reduplication: Repetition of the same syllable. Example: Many "baby talk" words are reduplicated, such as "boo-boo," "pee-pee," "mama," and the like.

Rhyme: The remainder of the syllable following the onset. Typically includes a nucleus (usually a vowel) and a coda (a consonant).

Rhythmic stereotypies: Rhythmic movements of body parts produced repeatedly, as in rocking on all fours, banging with two hands in sync, kicking with two feet in sync, and babbling.

Segmentation: The ability to break a whole into its component parts. Specifically, the ability to recognize the parts of a sentence (i.e., the words), a word (i.e., the syllables), or a syllable (i.e., the onset and rhyme or the individual phonemes).

Sensorimotor feedback loops: Neural connections, such as stretch receptors, through which the motor system gets updated concerning the state of the body or certain substructures.

Sensory integration: "The brain's ability to interpret and organize information from the senses" (Nicolisi, Harryman, & Kresheck, 1996, p. 245).

Sentence stress: Stress (in English, characterized by higher pitch and intensity with longer duration) on a particular word or phrase within a sentence for emphasis. Example: The implications of "*He* didn't steal the jewels" versus "He didn't *steal* the jewels" are very different.

Sequenced play routines: Ability to pretend using play routines that have a plot or a theme.

Soft neurological signs: Mild indicators of neurological disorder or difference, such as immature reflexes.

Stopping: Production of a target speech sound that is not a stop as a stop; usually applies to fricatives. Example: "Fish" pronounced as [pɪt] contains two instances of stopping of fricatives.

Stuffing: The overfilling of the mouth when eating, often for the increased sensory feedback provided.

Supraglottal: Produced via shaping or constriction of the vocal tract above the glottis. All English consonants and vowels, with the exception of [h] and [ʔ] (glottal stop), are supraglottal.

Suprasegmental: A phonological feature that spreads over more than just one sound segment. Includes prosody and also word-level patterns, such as consonant harmony.

Syllable: "A fundamental but elusive unit in phonology" (Trask, 1997, p. 214). Must include a nucleus (typically a vowel; sometimes a resonant consonant); may include an onset (initial consonant or cluster) and/or a coda (a final consonant or cluster).

Symptom complex: *See* Syndrome.

Syndrome: Cluster of symptoms with a common underlying deficit. No one symptom must be present in order for the syndrome to be identified; rather, it is the number and pattern of symptoms that indicates the appropriateness of the diagnosis.

Synthesis: "The combination of separate elements into a complex whole" (Morehead, 1995, p. 664).

Tactile stimulation: Generation of a response via the sense of touch.

Telegraphic speech: A stage in language development in which the child omits function words, producing sentences made up primarily of content words that therefore sound like telegrams. Example: "Me no want spinach."

Touch cues: Tactile stimulation to parts of the face and neck (by either the speech-language pathologist or the client) to facilitate the speaker's production of certain speech sounds. Example: The child's upper lip is touched to cue her or him to produce a bilabial sound.

"True" consonant: Any consonant other than a glottal ([h] or [ʔ]) or a glide ([w] or [j]).

Undershoot: Movement of a part of the body that is extended to less of a degree than was intended or is appropriate for accurate articulation.

Unitary disorder: A disorder characterized by a specific list of symptoms, all of which must be present in order for the disorder to be diagnosed.

Unstressed syllable augmentation: Production of a target unstressed syllable with a vowel that is more salient than in the target. For example, the pronunciation of "about" as [eɪbɑʊt] illustrates augmentation of the first syllable (i.e., the [ə] is replaced with a full diphthong).

Unstressed syllable deletion: The omission of a weak syllable in a word. Example: "about" pronounced as [bɑʊt].

Variegated babble: A type of prelinguistic vocalization in which a variety of consonants is produced rhythmically.

Velopharyngeal insufficiency: Inability to raise the soft palate enough to close off the velopharyngeal port and prevent leakage of air or food/drink into the nasal cavity.

Vocal play: A type of prelinguistic vocalization in which the child explores her or his vocal capacities in a primarily non-speech-like way, for example, by producing screeches, whispers, raspberries, tongue clicks, and so on.

Voicing errors: Production of targeted voiceless sounds as voiced or vice versa.

Volitional: Deliberately planned; not automatic, as in the production of a novel sentence.

Vowel deviation: Inappropriate production of a target vowel.

Vowel triangle: The set of vowels lying at the edges of the functional vowel space within the oral cavity: [i] (high front), [ɑ] (low back), [u] (high back).

Word stress: Stress (marked in English by higher pitch and intensity plus longer duration) on a particular syllable within a word. May be lexical, (i.e., always the same on a given word, such as "ra*vi*øli") or grammatical (e.g., the stress pattern differentiates a noun from a verb as in "*con*trast" versus "con*trast*").

REFERENCES

American Speech-Language-Hearing Association. (2001). *2001 Omnibus survey: Caseload reports: SLP*. Rockville, MD: ASHA.

Aram, D. (1984). Assessment and treatment of developmental apraxia. *Seminars in Speech and Language, 5*(2).

Ayres, A. J. (1985). *Developmental dyspraxia and adult-onset apraxia*. Torrance, CA: Sensory Integration International.

Bahr, D. C. (2001). *Oral motor assessment and treatment: Ages and stages*. Needham Heights, MA: Allyn & Bacon.

Bankson, N. (1990). *Bankson Language Screening Test: BLT-2*. Austin, TX: Pro-Ed.

Bankson, N. W., & Bernthal, J. E. (1990). *Bankson–Bernthal Test of Phonology (BB-TOP)*. Chicago: Riverside.

Bashir, A., Grahamjones, F., & Bostwick, R. (1984). A touch-cue method of therapy for developmental verbal apraxia. *Seminars in Speech and Language, 5*(2), 127–137.

Bernthal, J. E., & Bankson, N. W. (1998). *Articulation and phonological disorders* (4th ed.). Needham Heights, MA: Allyn & Bacon.

Bleile, K. M. (1995). *Manual of articulation and phonological disorders: Infancy through adulthood*. Clifton Park, NY: Singular.

Boshart, C. A. (1998). *Oral-motor analysis and remediation techniques*. Temecula, CA: Speech Dynamics.

Boynton, S. (1984). *Blue hat, green hat*. New York: Simon & Schuster.

Bridgeman, E., & Snowling, M. (1988). The perception of phoneme sequence: A comparison of dyspraxic and normal children. *British Journal of Disorders of Communication, 23*, 245–252.

Bzoch, K. R., & League, R. (1991). *Receptive-Expressive Emergent Language Scale* (2nd ed.). Austin, TX: Pro-Ed.

Carrow, E. (1974). *Carrow Elicited Language Inventory*. Austin, TX: Learning Concepts.

Carrow-Woolfolk, E. (1999). *Test for Auditory Comprehension of Language: TACL-3* (3rd ed.). Austin, TX: Pro-Ed.

Caruso, A. J., & Strand, E. A. (1999). *Clinical management of motor speech disorders in children*. New York: Thieme.

Chin, S., & Dinnsen, D. (1992). Consonant clusters in disordered speech:

Constraints and correspondence patterns. *Journal of Child Language, 19,* 259–285.

Chumpelik, D. (1984). The prompt system of therapy: Theoretical framework and applications for developmental apraxia of speech. *Seminars in Speech and Language, 5,* 139–153.

Cornett, R. (1972). *Cued speech parent training and follow-up program.* Washington, DC: Bureau of Education for Handicapped, DHEW 96; cited by Hall, Jordan, & Robin (1993) and Square (1999).

Crary, M. (1984). A neurolinguistic perspective on developmental verbal dyspraxia. *Journal of Communication Disorders, 9,* 33–49.

———. (1993). *Developmental motor speech disorders.* Clifton Park, NY: Singular.

Crystal, D. (1981). *Clinical linguistics.* Vienna: Springer-Verlag.

Crystal, D., Fletcher, P., & Garman, M. (1976). *The grammatical analysis of language disability: A procedure for assessment and intervention.* London: Edward Arnold.

Cunningham, P. (1996). *Phonics they use.* Glenview, IL: Harper Collins College Publishers.

Davis, B. L., Jakielski, K. J., & Marquardt, T. P. (1998). Developmental apraxia of speech: Determiners of differential diagnosis. *Clinical Linguistics & Phonetics, 12*(1), 25–45.

Davis, B. L., & MacNeilage, P. (1995). The articulatory basis of babbling. *Journal of Speech and Hearing Research, 38,* 1199–1211.

Davis, B. L., & Velleman, S. L. (2000). Differential diagnosis and treatment of developmental apraxia of speech in infants and toddlers. *Infant-Toddler Intervention, 10*(3), 177–192.

Dore, J. (1975). Holophrases, speech acts, and language universals. *Journal of Child Language, 2,* 21–40.

Dore, J., Franklin, M. B., Miller, R. T., & Ramer, A. L. H. (1976). Transitional phenomena in early language acquisition. *Journal of Child Language, 3,* 13–28.

Dunn, L. M., & Dunn, L. M. (1997). *PPVT-III: Peabody Picture Vocabulary Test.* Circle Pines, MN: American Guidance Systems.

Ekelman, B. L., & Aram, D. M. (1983). Syntactic findings in developmental verbal apraxia. *Journal of Communication Disorders, 16,* 237–250.

Fenson, L., Dale, P. S., Reznick, J. S., Thal, D., Bates, E., Hartung, J. P., Pethick, S., & Reilly, J. S. (1993). *MacArthur Communicative Development Inventories.* Clifton Park, NY: Singular.

Fisher, H. B., & Logemann, J. A. (1971). *The Fisher–Logemann Test of Articulation Competence.* Boston: Houghton Mifflin.

Fokes, J. (1976). *Fokes Sentence Builder.* Boston, MA: Teaching Resources Corporation.

Forrest, K. (2002). Are oral-motor exercises useful in the treatment of phonological/articulatory disorders? *Seminars in Speech and Language, 23*(1), 15–26.

Frederickson, N., Frith, U., & Reason, R. (1997). *Phonological Assessment Battery.* Windsor, Berks, UK: NFER-NELSON.

Frick, S., Frick, R., Oetter, P., & Richter, E. W. (1999). *Out of the mouths of babes: Discovering the developmental significance of the mouth.* New York: Psychological Corporation.

Frost, L. A., & Bondy, A. S. (1994). *The Picture Exchange Communication System (PECS) training manual.* Newark, DE: Pyramid Educational Consultants.

Fudala, J. B., & Reynolds, W. M. (1991). *Arizona Articulation Proficiency Scale* (2nd ed.). Los Angeles: Western Psychological Corporation.

Gardner, M. F. (2000a). *The Expressive One-Word Picture Vocabulary Test* (2000 ed.). Novato, CA: Academic Therapy Publications.

———. (2000b). *The Receptive One-Word Picture Vocabulary Test* (2000 ed.). Novato, CA: Academic Therapy Publications.

Gaskins, I. W., Downer, M. A., & Gaskins, R. W. (1986). *Introduction to the Benchmark School word identification/vocabulary development program.* Media, PA: Benchmark.

Gerken, L. A. (1991). The metrical basis for children's subjectless sentences. *Journal of Memory and Language, 30,* 431–451.

———. (1994a). A metrical template account of children's weak syllable omissions from multisyllabic words. *Journal of Child Language, 21*(3), 565–584.

———. (1994b). Young children's representation of prosodic structure: Evidence from English-speakers' weak syllable omissions. *Journal of Memory and Language, 33,* 19–38.

Gerken, L., & McIntosh, B. J. (1993). The interplay of function morphemes and prosody in early language. *Developmental Psychology, 29,* 448–457.

German, D. J. (2000). *Test of Word Finding - 2* (3rd ed.). Austin, TX: Pro-Ed.

Goldman, R., & Fristoe, M. (2000). *Goldman Fristoe Test of Articulation: GFTA-2* (2nd ed.). Chicago: Applied Symbolix.

Goldstein, B. (2000). *Cultural and linguistic diversity resource guide for speech-language pathologists.* Clifton Park, NY: Singular.

Goldsworthy, C. (1982). *Multilevel Informal Language Inventory: MILI.* Columbus, OH: Merrill.

Gordon-Brannan, M. (1994). Assessing intelligibility: Children's expressive phonologies. *Topics in Language Disorders, 14,* 17–25.

Goswami, U., & Bryant, P. (1990). *Phonological skills and learning to read.* East Sussex, UK: Erlbaum.

Gretz, S. (1998). Literacy development & children with apraxia of speech. Available 3/01 at http://www.apraxia-kids.org/literacy/literacy.html.

Grunwell, P. (1981). *The nature of phonological disability in children.* London: Academic.

———. (1985). *Phonological Assessment of Child Speech (PACS).* Scarborough, Ontario, Canada: Nelson Thomson Learning.

———. (1991). Developmental phonological disorders from a clinical-linguistic perspective. In M. S. Yavas (Ed.), *Phonological disorders in children: Theory, research and practice* (pp. 37–64). New York: Routledge.

———. (1993). Assessment of articulation and phonology. In J. R. Beech & L. Harding with D. Hilton-Jones (Eds.), *Assessment in speech and language therapy* (pp. 49–67). New York: Routledge.

Hall, P. K. (1989). The occurrence of developmental apraxia of speech in a mild articulation disorder: A case study. *Journal of Communication Disorders, 22,* 265–276.

Hall, P., Jordan, L., & Robin, D. (1993). *Developmental apraxia of speech.* Austin, TX: Pro-Ed.

Hargrove, P., & McGarr, G. (1994). *Prosody management of communication disorders.* Clifton Park, NY: Singular.

Hayden, D. A., & Square, P. A. (1994). Motor speech treatment hierarchy: A systems approach. *Clinics in Communication Disorders, 4,* 162–174.

———. (1999). *VMPAC: Verbal Motor Production Assessment for Children.* San Antonio: Psychological Corporation.

Haynes, S. (1985). Developmental apraxia of speech: Symptoms and treatment. In D. Johns (Ed.), *Clinical management of neurogenic communication disorders* (pp. 259–266). Boston: Little, Brown.

Hedrick, D., Prather, E., & Tobin, A. (1984). *Sequenced Inventory of Communication Development.* Seattle: University of Washington Press.

Hegde, M. N. (1997). *Pocketguide to assessment in speech-language pathology.* Clifton Park, NY: Singular.

Helfrich-Miller, K. (1984). Melodic intonation therapy with developmentally apraxic children. *Seminars in Speech and Language, 5*(2), 119–126.

Hempenstall, K. (1999). Beginning reading instruction: The role of phonemic awareness and phonics. *1999 Successful Learning Conference* University of Western Sydney. Available 3/01 at http://www.rmit.edu.au/departments/ps/staffpgs/hempenart/1999.htm.

Hill, E. (1980). *Where's Spot?* New York: Putnam.

Hodson, B. (1986). *The Assessment of Phonological Processes-Revised.* Austin, TX: Pro-Ed.

Hodson, B. W., & Paden, E. P. (1991). *Targeting intelligible speech: A phonological approach to remediation* (2nd ed.). Austin, TX: Pro-Ed.

Hresko, W. P., Reid, D. K., & Hammill, D. (1999). *Test of Early Language Development: TELD-3* (3rd ed.). Austin, TX: Pro-Ed.

Ingram, D. (1981). *Procedures for the Phonological Analysis of Children's Language.* Baltimore: University Park Press.

———. (1990). *Phonological disability in children* (2nd ed.). Clifton Park, NY: Singular.

International Phonetic Association. (1999). *Handbook of the International Phonetic Association.* Cambridge, UK: Cambridge University Press.

Jordan, L. S. (1988). Gestures for cuing phonemes in verbal apraxia: A case study. Paper presented at the American Speech-Language-Hearing Association meeting, Boston, MA. Cited by Hall, Jordan, & Robin (1993).

Jordan, L. S. (1991). Treating apraxia of speech. Paper presented at the Midwest Aphasiology Conference, Iowa City. Cited by Hall, Jordan, & Robin, (1993).

Kaufman, N. (1995). *Kaufman Speech Praxis Test for Children.* Detroit: Wayne State University Press.

———. (1998). *Speech Praxis Treatment Kit for Children.* Gaylord, MI: Northern Speech Services.

———. (2001). *Speech Praxis Treatment Kit for Children-2.* Gaylord, MI: Northern Speech Services.

Kehoe, M. (1995). *An investigation of rhythmic processes in English-speaking children's word productions.* Unpublished doctoral dissertation, University of Washington.

———. (1997). Stress error patterns in English-speaking children's word productions. *Clinical Linguistics & Phonetics, 11*(5), 389–409.

Kehoe, M., & Stoel-Gammon, C. (1997a). The acquisition of prosodic structure: An investigation of current accounts of children's prosodic development. *Language, 73*(1), 113–144.

———. (1997b). Truncation patterns in English-speaking children's word productions. *Journal of Speech Language and Hearing Research, 40*(3), 526–541.

Kent, R. D. (Ed.). (1992). *Intelligibility in speech disorders.* Philadelphia: John Benjamins.

Kent, R. D., & Bauer, H. R. (1985). Vocalizations of one-year-olds. *Journal of Child Language, 12,* 491–526.

Khan, L., & Lewis, N. (1986). *Khan–Lewis Phonological Analysis.* Circle Pines, MN: American Guidance Service.

Kirkpatrick, J., Stohr, P., & Kimbrough, D. (1990). *Moving Across Syllables.* Tucson, AZ: Communication Skill Builders.

Klick, S. L. (1984). Adapted cueing technique for use in treatment of dyspraxia. *Speech Language and Hearing Services in the Schools, 16,* 256–259. Cited by Square (1999).

Klick, S. L. (1994). Adapted cuing technique: Faciliitating sequential phoneme production. *Clinics in Communication Disorders, 4,* 183–189; cited by Square (1999)

Koopmans-van Beinum, F. J., & van der Stelt, J. M. (1986). Early stages in the development of speech movements. In B. Lindbolm & R. Zetterstrom (Eds.), *Precursors of early speech.* New York: Stockton.

Kresheck, J. D., & Werner, E. O. (1989). *Structured Photographic Articulation Test Featuring Dudsberry.* Sandwich, IL: Janelle Publications.

Lee, L. (1974). *Developmental sentence analysis.* Evanston, IL: Northwestern University Press.

Leonard, L. B., & McGregor, K. K. (1991). Unusual phonological patterns and their underlying representations: A case study. *Journal of Child Language, 18*(2), 261–272.

Lindamood, C., & Lindamood, P. (1979). *Lindamood Auditory Conceptualization Test-Revised: LAC.* Allen, TX: DLM.

———. (1998). *Lindamood® Phoneme Sequencing Program for Reading, Spelling, and Speech* (3rd ed.). San Luis Obispo, CA: Gander Educational Publishing.

Linder, T. W. (1993a). *Transdisciplinary Play-Based Assessment: TPBA.* Baltimore: Brookes.

Linder, T. W. (1993b). *Transdisciplinary Play-Based Assessment: TPBA.* Baltimore: Brookes.

Lippkey, B. A., Dickey, S. E., Selmar, J. W., & Soder, A. L. (1997). *Photo Articulation Test* (3rd ed.). Austin, TX: Pro-Ed.

Long, S., & Fey, M. (1993). *Computerized Profiling.* San Diego: Singular.

Love, R. J. (1992). *Childhood motor speech disability.* New York: Macmillan.

———. (2000). *Childhood motor speech disability* (2nd ed.). Boston: Allyn & Bacon.

Lowe, R. J. (1993). *Speech-language pathology & related professions in the schools.* Needham Heights, MA: Allyn & Bacon.

———. (1995). *Assessment Link between Phonology and Articulation-Revised (ALPHA-R).* Mifflinville, PA: Alpha Speech and Language Resources, Box 322.

Lowe, M., & Costello, A. (1976). *The Symbolic Play Test.* London: National Foundation of Educational Research.

Lund, N., & Duchan, J. (1988). *Assessing children's language in naturalistic contexts.* Englewood Cliffs, NJ: PrenticeHall.

Mackie, E. (1996a). *Oral-motor activities for school-aged children.* East Moline, IL: LinguiSystems.

———. (1996b). *Oral-motor activities for young children.* East Moline, IL: LinguiSystems.

MacNeilage, P. F., & Davis, B. L. (1990). Acquisition of speech production: Frames, then content. In M. Geannerod (Ed.), *Motor representation and control* (pp. 453–475). Hillsdale, NJ: Erlbaum.

Marion, M. J., Sussman, H. M., & Marquardt, T. P. (1993). The perception and production of rhyme in normal and developmentally apraxic children. *Journal of Communication Disorders, 26,* 129–160.

Marquardt, T., & Sussman, H. (1991). Developmental apraxia of speech: Theory and practice. In D. Vogel & M. Cannito (Eds.), *Treating disordered speech motor control* (pp. 341–390). Austin, TX: Pro-Ed.

Marquardt, T. P., Sussman, H. M., Snow, T., & Jacks, A. (2002). The integrity of the syllable in developmental apraxia of speech. *Journal of Communication Disorders, 35,* 31–49.

Martin, B. (1996). *Brown bear, brown bear, what do you see?* New York: Henry Holt.

Mayer, M. (1983). *I was so mad.* New York: Golden Books.

McCabe, P., Rosenthal, J. B., & McLeod, S. (1998). Features of developmental dyspraxia in the general speech-impaired population? *Clinical Lingusitics and Phonetics, 12*(2), 105–126.

McCathren, R., Warren, S., & Yoder, P. (1996). Prelinguistic predictors of later language development. In K. Cole, P. Dale, & D. Thal (Eds.), *Assessment of communication and language.* Baltimore: Brookes.

Miller, J., & Chapman, R. (1995). *SALT: Systematic Analysis of Language Transcripts.* Madison: Language Analysis Laboratory, University of Wisconsin.

Moreau, M. R., & Fidrych-Puzzo, H. (1994). *How to use the Story Grammar Marker.* Easthampton, MA: Discourse Skills Productions.

Morehead, P. D. (Ed.). (1995). *The new American Webster handy college dictionary* (3rd ed.). New York: Penguin.

Morris, S. E. (1993). *The development of oral-motor skills in children receiving non-oral feedings.* Faber, VA: New Visions.

———. (1997a). Feeding and speech relationships. Available 2/24/ 01 at http://www.new-vis.com/fym/papers/p-feed8.htm.

———. (1997b). Mouth toys open the sensory doorway. Available 2/24/01 at http://www.newvis.com/fym/papers/p-feed1.htm.

———. (1997c). Stuffing. Available 2/24/ 01 at http://www.new-vis.com/fym/papers/p-feed11.htm.

Most, B. (1996). *Cock-a-doodle-moo!* New York: Harcourt Brace.

———. (1997a). *Moo ha.* New York: Harcourt Brace.

———. (1997b). *Oink ha.* New York: Harcourt Brace.

Netsell, R. (1981). The acquisition of speech motor control: A perspective with directions for research. In R. Stark (Ed.), *Language behavior in infancy and early childhood* (pp. 127–153). Elsevier North Holland.

Newcomer, P. L., & Hammill, D. D. (1997). *Test of Language Development-Primary: TOLD-P:3.* New York: Psychological Corporation.

Nicolich, L. (1977). Beyond sensorimotor intelligence: Assessment of symbolic maturity through analysis of pretend play. *Merrill Palmer Quarterly, 23,* 89–101.

Nicolisi, L., Harryman, E., & Kresheck, J. (1996). *Terminology of communication disorders: Speech-language-hearing* (4th ed.). Baltimore: Williams & Wilkins.

Oetter, P., Richter, E., & Frick, S. (1995). *MORE: Integrating the mouth with sensory and postural functions* (2nd ed.). Hugo, MN: P.D.P.

Oller, D. K. (1986). Metaphonology and infant vocalizations. In B. Lindblom & R. Zetterstrom (Eds.), *Precursors of early speech.* New York: Stockton.

Olswang, L., Stoel-Gammon, C., Coggins, T., & Carpenter, R. (1987). *Assessing prelinguistic and early linguistic behaviors in developmentally young children.* Seattle: University of Washington Press.

Owens, R. E., Jr. (1996). *Language development: An introduction.* Needham Heights, MA: Allyn & Bacon.

Pehrsson, R. S., & Robinson, H. A. (1985). *The semantic organizer approach to writing and reading instruction.* Rockville, MD: Aspen.

Peppé, S., & Wells, B. (2001). *Profiling Elements of Prosodic Systems—Children (PEPS-C).* Test under development.

Proctor, A. (1989). Stages of normal non-cry vocal development in infancy: A protocol for assessment. *Topics in Language Disorders, 10*(1), 26–42.

Purves, D., Augustine, G. J., Fitzpatrick, D., Katz, L. C., LaManita, A.-S., & McNamara, J. O. (Eds.) (1997) *Neuroscience.* Sunderland, MA: Sinauer Associates.

Retherford, K. (1993). *Guide to analysis of language transcripts.* Eau Claire, WI: Thinking Publications.

Reynell, J. (1969). *Reynell Developmental Language Scales.* Buckinghamshire, UK: National Foundation for Educational Research in England and Wales.

Ripley, K., Daines, B., & Barrett, J. (1997). *Dyspraxia: A guide for teachers and parents.* London: David Fulton.

Robbins, J., & Klee, T. (1987). Clinical assessment of oropharyngeal motor development in young children. *Journal of Speech and Hearing Disorders, 52,* 271–277.

Robertson, C., & Salter, W. (1997). *The Phonological Awareness Test.* East Moline, IL: LinguiSystems.

Robin, D. A. (1992). Developmental apraxia of speech: Just another motor problem. *American Journal of Speech-Language Pathology, 1,* 19–22.

Rosenbek, J., Hansen, R., Baughman, C., & Lemme, M. (1974). Treatment of developmental apraxia of speech. *Language, Speech, and Hearing Services in the Schools, 5,* 13–22; cited by Crary (1993).

Rosenbek, J., & Wertz, R. (1972). A review of 50 cases of developmental apraxia of speech. *Language Speech and Hearing Services in the Schools, 3,* 23–30.

Schwartz, R. G., & Goffman, L. (1995). Metrical patterns of words and production accuracy. *Journal of Speech and Hearing Research, 38*(4), 876–888.

Secord, W. (1981). *Test of Minimal Articulation Competence (T-MAC).* San Antonio: Psychological Corporation.

Secord, W. A., & Shine, R. E. (1997). *Secord Contextual Articulation Tests.* Sedona, AZ: Red Rock Educational Publications.

Semel, E., Wiig, E. H., & Secord, W. (1992). *Clinical Evaluation of Language Fundamentals — Preschool (CELF-P).* New York: Psychological Corporation.

———. (1995). *Clinical Evaluation of Language Fundamentals (CELF)* (3rd ed.). New York: Psychological Corporation.

Seuss, D. (1996). *There's a wocket in my pocket.* New York: Random House.

Shattuck-Hufnagel, S. (1982). Three kinds of speech error evidence for the role of grammatical elements in processing. In L. Obler & L. Menn (Eds.), *Exceptional language and linguistics.* New York: Academic Press.

————. (1992). The role of word structure in segmental serial ordering. *Cognition, 42,* 213–259.

————. (1994). Stress shift and early pitch accent placement in lexical items in American English. *Journal of Phonetics, 22,* 357–388.

————. (1996). A prosody tutorial for investigators of auditory sentence processing. *Journal of Psycholinguistic Research, 25*(2), 193–247.

Shipley, K. G., & McAfee, J. G. (1992). *Assessment in speech-language pathology.* Clifton Park, NY: Singular.

Shriberg, L. D. (1986). *PEPPER: Programs to examine phonetic and phonologic evaluation records.* Hillsdale, NJ: Erlbaum.

Shriberg, L. D., Aram, D. M., & Kwiatkowski, J. (1997a). Developmental apraxia of speech: I. Descriptive and theoretical perspectives. *Journal of Speech Language and Hearing Research, 40*(2), 273–285.

————. (1997b). Developmental apraxia of speech: II. Toward a diagnostic marker. *Journal of Speech Language and Hearing Research,* 40(2), 286–312.

————. (1997c). Developmental apraxia of speech: III. A subtype marked by inappropriate stress. *Journal of Speech Language and Hearing Research,* 40(2), 313–337.

————, L. D., & Kent, R. D. (1995). *Clinical phonetics* (2nd ed.). Boston: Allyn & Bacon.

Shriberg, L. D., & Kwiatkowski, J. (1980). *Natural Process Analysis (NPA).* New York: Wiley.

————. (1982). Phonological disorders I: A diagnostic classification system. *Journal of Speech and Hearing Disorders, 47,* 226–241.

————. (1983). Computer-assisted natural process analysis (NPA): Recent issues and data. *Seminars in Speech and Language, 4,* 397–406.

Shriberg, L. D., Kwiatkowski, J., & Rasmussen, C. (1990). *Prosody-Voice Screening Profile.* Tucson, AZ: Communication Skill Builders.

Shriberg, L. D., Tomblin, J. B., & McSweeny, J. L. (1999). Prevalence of speech delay in 6-year-old children and comorbidity with language impairment. *Journal of Speech, Language, and Hearing Research, 41*(6), 1461–1481.

Shulman, B. (1986). *Test of Pragmatic Skills, Revised.* Tucson, AZ: Communication Skill Builders.

Smit, A. B., Hand, L., Freilinger, J. J., Bernthal, J. E., & Bird, A. (1990). The Iowa articulation norms project and its Nebraska replication. *Journal of Speech and Hearing Disorders, 55*(4), 779–798.

Smith, B. L., Brown-Sweeney, S., & Stoel-Gammon, C. (1989). A quantitative analysis of reduplicated and variegated babbling. *First Language, 9,* 175–190.

Smith, P. K., & Engel, B. J. (1984). *Melodic apraxia training.* Tucson, AZ: Communication Skill Builders. Cited by Square (1999).

Snowling, M., & Stackhouse, J. (1983). Spelling performance of children with developmental verbal dyspraxia. *Developmental Medicine and Child Neurology, 25,* 430–437.

Square, P. A. (1994). Treatment approaches for developmental apraxia of speech. *Clinics in Communication Disorders, 4,* 151–161.

———. (1999). Treatment of developmental apraxia of speech: Tactile-kinesthetic, rhythmic, and gestural approaches. In A. J. Caruso & E. A. Strand (Eds.), *Clinical management of motor speech disorders in children* (pp. 149–186). New York: Thieme.

Stackhouse, J. (1982). An investigation of reading and spelling performance in speech disordered children. *British Journal of Disorders of Communication, 17,* 52–59.

———. (1992). Developmental verbal dyspraxia: A longitudinal case study. In R. Campbell (Ed.), *Mental lives* (pp. 84–98). Cambridge, MA: Blackwell.

———. (1997). Phonological awareness: Connecting speech and literacy problems. In B. W. Hodson & M. L. Edwards (Eds.), *Perspectives in applied phonology* (pp. 157–196). Gaithersburg, MD: Aspen.

Stackhouse, J., & Wells, B. (1997). *Children's speech and literacy difficulties: A psycholinguistic framework.* London: Whurr.

Stackhouse, J., & Wells, B. (Ed.). (2000). *Children's speech and literacy difficulties: Identification and intervention: Book II.* London: Whurr.

Stackhouse, J., Wells, B., Pascoe, M., & Rees, R. (2002). From phonological therapy to phonological awareness. *Seminars in Speech and Language, 23*(1), 27–42.

Stark, R., Bernstein, L., & Demorest, M. (1993). Vocal communication in the first 18 months of life. *Journal of Speech and Hearing Research, 36,* 548–558.

Stickler, K. R. (1987). *Guide to analysis of language transcripts.* Eau Claire, WI: Thinking Publications.

Stoel-Gammon, C. (1987). Phonological skills of 2-year-olds. *Language Speech and Hearing Services in the Schools, 18,* 323–329.

———. (1988). Prelinguistic vocalizations of hearing-impaired and normally hearing subjects: A comparison of consonantal inventories. *Journal of Speech and Hearing Disorders, 53*(3), 302–315.

———. (1989). Prespeech and early speech development of two late talkers. *First Language, 9,* 207–224.

———. (1992). Prelinguistic vocal development: Measurement and predictions. In C. A. Ferguson, L. Menn, & C. Stoel-Gammon (Eds.), *Phonological development: Models, research, and implications* (pp. 439–456). Monkton, MD: York.

Stoel-Gammon, C., & Cooper, J. A. (1984). Patterns of early lexical and phonological development. *Journal of Child Language, 11,* 247–271.

Stoel-Gammon, C., & Stone, J. R. (1991). Assessing phonology in young children. *Clinics in Communication Disorders, 1*(2), 25–39.

Stoel-Gammon, C., Stone-Goldman, J & Glaspey, A. (2002). Pattern-bas approaches to phonological thera *Seminars in Speech and Langu 23*(1), 3–14.

Strand, E. A., & McCauley, R. J. (Assessment procedures for tre planning in children with ph and motor speech disorders. Caruso & E. A. Strand (Eds.) management of motor speech in children (pp. 73–107). Thieme.

Strand, E. A., & Skinder, A. (1999). Treatment of developmental apraxia of speech: Integral stimulation methods. In A. J. Caruso & E. A. Strand (Eds.), *Clinical management of motor speech disorders in children* (pp. 109–148). New York: Thieme.

Strand, K. (1997). Oral motor function assessment. Unpublished assessment protocol.

Strub, R. L., & Black, F. W. (1981). *Organic brain syndromes: An introduction to neurobehavioral disorders.* Philadelphia: Davis.

Templin, M., & Darley, F. (1969). *The Templin-Darley Tests of Articulation.* Iowa City: Bureau of Educational Research and Service, University of Iowa.

Thal, D., & Tobias, S. (1992). Communicative gestures in children with delayed onset of oral expressive vocabulary. *Journal of Speech and Hearing Research, 35,* 1281–1289.

Thelen, E. (1981). Rhythmical behavior in infancy: An ethological perspective. *Developmental Psychology, 17,* 237–257.

Torgesen, J. K., & Bryant, B. R. (1994). *Test of Phonological Awareness.* Austin, TX: Pro-Ed.

Trask, R. L. (1997). *A student's dictionary of language and linguistics.* New York: St. Martin's.

Tyack, D., & Gottsleben, R. (1974). *Language sampling, analysis, and training: A handbook for teachers and clinicians.* Palo Alto, CA: Consulting Psychologists.

___er, A. A. (2002). Language-based ___ervention for phonological disor-___. *Seminars in Speech and Lan-___ e, 23*(1), 69–82.

___ S. L. (1994). The interaction of ___s and phonology in develop-

mental verbal dyspraxia: Two case studies. *Clinics in Communication Disorders, 4*(1), 67–78.

_____. (1996). Metathesis highlights feature-by-position constraints. In B. Bernhardt, J. Gilbert, & D. Ingram (Eds.), *Proceedings of the UBC International Conference on Phonological Acquisition* (pp. 173–186). Somerville, MA: Cascadilla.

_____. (1998). *Making phonology functional: What do I do first?* Boston: Butterworth-Heinemann.

_____. (2002). Phonotactic therapy. *Seminars in Speech and Language, 23*(1), 43–56.

_____. S. L., & Shriberg, L. D. (1999). Metrical analysis of children with suspected developmental apraxia of speech and inappropriate stress. *Journal of Speech Language and Hearing Research, 42*(6), 1444–1460.

Velleman, S., & Strand, K. (1994). Developmental verbal dyspraxia. In J. E. Bernthal & N. W. Bankson (Eds.), *Child phonology: Characteristics, assessment, and intervention with special populations* (pp. 110–139). New York: Thieme.

_____. (1998). Dynamic remediation strategies for children with developmental verbal dyspraxia. Videoteleconference available from the American Speech-Language-Hearing Association.

Vihman, M., Ferguson, C., & Elbert, M. (1986). Phonological development from babbling to speech: Common tendencies and individual differences. *Applied Psycholinguistics, 7,* 3–40.

Vihman, M. M., & Greenlee, M. (1987). Individual differences in phonological development: Ages one and three years. *Journal of Speech and Hearing Research, 30,* 503–521.

Vihman, M. M., Macken, M. A., Miller, R., Simmons, H., & Miller, J. (1985). From babbling to speech: A reassessment of the continuity issue. *Language, 61,* 395–443.

Vihman, M. M., & Miller, R. (1988). Words and babble at the threshold of lexical acquisition. In M. D. Smith & J. L. Locke (Eds.), *The emergent lexicon: The child's development of a linguistic vocabulary* (pp. 151–183). New York: Academic.

Wallace, G., & Hammill, D. D. (1997). *Comprehensive Receptive and Expressive Vocabulary Test: CREVT.* Austin, TX: Pro-Ed.

Weiner, F. F. (1979). *Phonological Process Analysis.* Austin, TX: Pro-Ed.

Weiss, A. L. (2001). *Preschool language disorders: Resource guide.* Clifton Park, NY: Singular.

Wells, B., & Peppé, S. (2000). Intonation within a psycholinguistic framework. In J. Stackhouse & B. Wells (Eds.), *Children's speech and literacy difficulties: Identification and Intervention: Book II.* London: Whurr.

Wells, B., & Peppé, S. (2001). Intonation abilities of children with speech and language impairments. Ms, University of Sheffield, UK.

Wells, B., Peppé, S., & Goulandris, N. (2001). Intonation development from five to thirteen. Ms, University of Sheffield, UK.

Wells, B., Peppé, S., & Vance, M. (1995). Linguistic assessment of prosody. In K. Grundy (Ed.), *Linguistics in clinical practice* (pp. 234–265). Clifton Park, NY: Singular.

Westby, C. (1980). Assessment of cognitive and language abilities through play. *Language, Speech, and Hearing Services in Schools, 11,* 154–168.

———. (1991). A scale for assessing children's pretend play. In C. Schaefer, K. Gitlin, & A. Sandgrund (Eds.). *Play diagnosis and assessment,* New York: Wiley.

Wetherby, A., Cain, D., Yonclas, D., & Walker, V. (1988). Analysis of intentional communication of normal children from the prelinguistic to the multiword stage. *Journal of Speech and Hearing Research, 31,* 240–252.

Wetherby, A., & Prizant, B. (1993). *Communication and Symbolic Behavior Scales.* Chicago: Riverside.

Wetherby, A., & Rodriguez, G. (1992). Measurement of communicative intentions in normally developing children during structured and unstructured contexts. *Journal of Speech and Hearing Research, 35,* 130–138.

Williams, R., Ingham, R. J., & Rosenthal, J. (1981). A further analysis for developmental apraxia of speech in children with defective articulation. *Journal of Speech and Hearing Research, 24,* 496–505.

Yoss, K., & Darley, F. (1974). Therapy in developmental apraxia of speech. *Language, Speech and Hearing Services in Schools, 5,* 23–31.

Young, E. H., & Stichfield-Hawk, S. (1955). *Moto-kinesthetic speech training therapy.* Stanford, CA: Stanford University Press. Cited by Square (1999).

Zachman, L., Hulsingh, R., Jorgensen, C., & Barrett, M. (1978). *Oral Language Sentence Imitation Test.* Moline, IL: Linguisystems.

Zimmerman, I. L., Steiner, V. G., & P. R. E. (1992). *Preschool Language - 3* (PLS-3). San Antonio: Communication Skill Builders.

INDEX

T

Thelen, E., 7
"Time to Sing," 73
training automaticity, 72–73
training motor-planning flexibility, 74–75
   and ability to anticipate articulatory change in
      phonetic sequences, 74
   and ability to produce repeated phonetic
      sequences, 74
   possible strategies, 75

U

undershoot, 15, 16
unitary disorder, 4

V

Velleman, S., 4, 8, 54, 55, 58, 61, 62, 72
velopharyngeal insufficiency, 16
Verbal Motor Production Assessment for Children
    (VMPAC / Hayden and Square), 17
Vocal Development Checklist Form, 19
vocal play, 19

W

Wells, B., 41
word(s), 5. *See also* blending; compound words
word stress, 17